Breaking Bread, Nourishing Connections

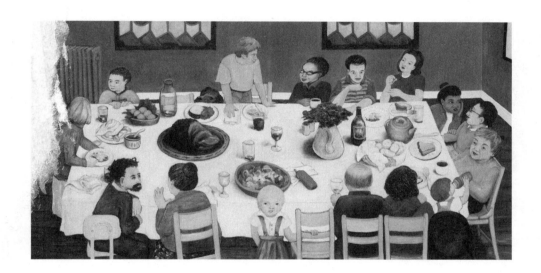

BREAKING BREAD, NOURISHING CONNECTIONS

People with and without Disabilities Together at Mealtime

by

Karin Melberg Schwier

and

Erin Schwier Stewart, O.T.D., OTR/L

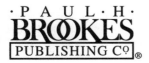
·P·A·U·L·H·
BROOKES
PUBLISHING C.®

Baltimore • London • Sydney

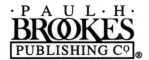

Paul H. Brookes Publishing Co.
Post Office Box 10624
Baltimore, Maryland 21285-0624

www.brookespublishing.com

"Paul H. Brookes Publishing Co." is a registered trademark of
Paul H. Brookes Publishing Co., Inc.

Typeset by Barton Matheson Willse & Worthington, Baltimore, Maryland.
Manufactured in the United States of America by Victor Graphics, Baltimore, Maryland.

The individuals featured in the vignettes in this book have kindly granted permission for their actual
names, stories, and photographs to be used. Pseudonyms have been used for other individuals and some
institutions.

The cover painting, "Gathering," was created expressly for this book by J. Spencer Schwier.

Recipe illustrations were provided courtesy of Elizabeth Boling.

"Recipe Box Letters, #5," by Michael Bradford, is from the book *Personal Effects* (2004), published by
Coteau Books, 401–2206 Dewdney Ave., Regina, SK S4R 1H3. http://www.coteaubooks.com
Used by permission of the publisher.

Excerpts on pp. 123–124 are from COMMUNITY AND GROWTH (revised Edition) by Jean Vanier,
Copyright © 1989 by Paulist Press, Paulist Press, Inc., New York/Mahwah, N.J. Used with permission.
www.paulistpress.com

The photo on p. 70 was taken by Dick Sobsey. The photo on p. 88 was taken by Robert Powell. The
photos on pp. 117, 125, 132, and 140 were taken by Beth Porter.

Library of Congress Cataloging-in-Publication Data

Schwier, Karin Melberg.
  Breaking bread, nourishing connections : people with and without disabilities together at mealtime /
by Karen Melberg Schwier and Erin Schwier Stewart.
    p.   cm.
  Includes bibliographical references and index.
  ISBN 1-55766-720-9 (pbk.)
  1. Cookery for people with disabilities.   I. Stewart, Erin Schwier.   II. Title.

TX652.S423   2005
641.5′631—dc22   2005001241

British Library Cataloguing in Publication data are available from the British Library.

For Mary Ervin Liming Schwier
"Momo"
1915–2004

Among my mother-in-law's happiest occasions were the rare times when her far-flung family gathered at her Florida table to enjoy her German potato salad, a good ham, baked creamed corn, and Jell-O salads. And she was always on a quest to bake the perfect pie. "If only we all lived close enough to have Sunday dinners together," she would say. We will always treasure those Sundays when we could.
—K.M.S.

For Dad and Karin, who taught me the importance of waffles on Sunday. To my husband Michael for his support from start to finish. And for my Momo. There wasn't anything a few Momo cookies couldn't fix.
—E.S.S.

v

Contents

About the Authors

Karin Melberg Schwier, Copestone Writing, 908 University Drive, Saskatoon, Saskatchewan, S7N 0K1, Canada (http://homepage.mac.com/karin.schwier/copestone), is an author and illustrator whose most noted works are about people with intellectual disabilities. Among her books are *Sexuality: Your Sons and Daughters with Intellectual Disabilities*, coauthored with Dave Hingsburger (Paul H. Brookes Publishing Co., 2000) and *Couples with Intellectual Disabilities Talk About Living and Loving* (Woodbine House, 1994). She is the stepparent of Jim, 30, a young man with an intellectual disability; co-author Erin Schwier Stewart, 28; and Benjamin, 24. Karin lives in Saskatoon with Jim and her husband Richard, a professor of education. They have a 24-year-old cat, Max, who prefers his food warm.

Erin Schwier Stewart, O.T.D, OTR/L, Box 880064, San Diego, California 92168 (eschwier@western.edu), received a doctorate in occupational therapy at the University of Southern California in 2003. She received a master's degree in occupational therapy from USC in 2002 and a bachelor of science degree from San Diego State University in 1999. She has a particular interest in disability advocacy in health policy. Currently a pediatric occupational therapist in private practice, she is also a senior policy fellow and occupational therapist at the Center for Disability Issues and the Health Professions, Western University of Health Sciences, Pomona, California. She is the sister of a young man with an intellectual disability. Erin lives in San Diego with her husband, Michael Stewart, who is in law enforcement, and their beagle, Nickels, who enjoys plastic sausages.

About the Illustrators

Elizabeth Boling (illustrated recipes, icons) (http://php.ucs.indiana.edu/~eboling/ and http://www.indiana.edu/~iirg/) is Associate Professor and Department Head of Indiana University's Department of Instructional Systems Technology. She teaches courses in instructional design and visual design. With a strong background in art, design, and computing, her approach is to integrate the two disciplines of instructional design and graphic design. She was formerly with Apple Computer, where she was Graphics and Animation Manager. Elizabeth conducted usability testing pilot sessions with people with disabilities and their families of all illustrated recipes in this book. Based on the feedback, adjustments improved the ease with which the instructions can be understood and followed. She is the friend of a young man with an intellectual disability and lives near Bloomington, Indiana.

J. Spencer Schwier (cover art) received a bachelor of fine arts in 1997 from the University of Cincinnati, with a specific interest in drawing and painting. His portfolio includes logos, murals, illustrations, photography, and paintings. He lives with his wife Nani, a social worker, and their three children in Lawrenceburg, Indiana, where he creates commissioned pieces. He has grown up around his father's restaurant business and is the cousin of a young man with an intellectual disability.

About the Project Advisors

Julie Hodges, Ph.D., RD, LDN, FADA, is a nutritionist/dietician and the Director of Health Care Services, Zartic. The author of several publications and presentations, she was an adjunct professor at Tulsa Medical College, Carson Newman College, and the University of Tennessee. She was a Major in the Medical Specialist Corps, United States Army Reserves. She has been a nutrition consultant with several residential facilities and develops food for people with difficulty chewing and swallowing and also for people with developmental disabilities. Her interest is fueled by a personal experience; her brother had multiple sclerosis. As his condition deteriorated, he went from eating like the rest of the family to having his food chopped, then ground, then puréed, until finally he ate through a tube. Julie saw how much the aromas, flavors and sharing of mealtime with family and friends meant to him. Julie provided the nutritional analysis for all recipes included in this book and reviewed the Tidbits section. She lives in Rome, Georgia.

Robert Perske is the author of best-selling books on building community with people who have disabilities, including *Circles of Friends: People with Disabilities and Their Friends Enrich the Lives of One Another* (Abingdon Press, 1988). He was an editor of the groundbreaking book, *Mealtimes for Severely and Profoundly Handicapped Persons* (University Park Press, 1977; Paul H. Brookes Publishing, Co., 1986 [re-release]). In recent years, Robert has focused his writing and advocacy energies on the criminal justice system. *Unequal Justice? What Can Happen When Persons with Retardation or Other Developmental Disabilities Encounter the Criminal Justice System* (Abingdon Press, 1991) and *Deadly Innocence?* (Abingdon Press, 1995). He is currently working on a collection of his works on this subject. Robert lives in Darien, Connecticut, with his wife, artist Martha Perske.

Richard A. Schwier, Ed.D., is Professor of Education, University of Saskatchewan. Richard is an instructional designer with a particular interest in the development of on-line communities. He is also the parent of a son with an intellectual disability. Richard learned meal preparation, presentation, and serving skills as an employee of Hook's Catering, Indianapolis, Indiana, in the 1970s while he attended Indiana University. An enthusiastic cook, he lives in Saskatoon, Saskatchewan.

Todd Zazelenchuk, Ed.D., is a designer and evaluator of human–machine interactions. He has worked as a schoolteacher, an instructional designer, and a consultant in both academia and industry. Originally from the prairies of western Canada, he has a doctorate in instructional technology from Indiana University. When asked to serve as an advisor, Todd responded, "What time is the first meal?" He is a member of a friendship network and a trustee for a man with an intellectual disability. He lives in St. Joseph, Michigan, and works as a human factors researcher for Whirlpool Corporation, where he is responsible for the quality of user interactions with all KitchenAid countertop appliances. Here, Todd gets to combine his research skills with his love for design, gadgets, cooking, and eating.

About the Contributors

CHAPTER AUTHORS

Bill Gaventa, M.Div., New Brunswick, New Jersey, serves as Director of Community and Congregational Supports at the Elizabeth M. Boggs Center on Developmental Disabilities, and Associate Professor, Robert Wood Johnson Medical School. The Center is part of the Robert Wood Johnson Medical School of the University of Medicine and Dentistry of New Jersey. Bill works on community supports, training for community services staff, and supervision of a program in clinical pastoral education. He also coordinates a training and technical assistance team for the New Jersey Self Determination Initiative, a statewide process now supporting approximately 300 individuals and their families. His publications experience includes serving as co-editor of the *Journal of Religion, Disability, and Health,* editor of two newsletters, and a columnist for *Insight,* the national newsletter of The Arc of the United States. He has served as Executive Secretary for the Religion and Spirituality Division of the American Association on Mental Retardation (AAMR) since 1985. He currently serves on the Board of Directors of the AAMR.

Barb Handahl, Faribault, Minnesota, has worked for the Department of Human Services for 32 years. She worked at the Faribault Regional Center from 1968 to 1991 in various lead worker positions both in the Residential and Day Program Services areas. Since 1991, she has worked at a Minnesota State Operated Community Services (MSOCS) Home in Faribault. She is committed to person-centered planning and is active in various roles. She currently is the co-chair of the Person-Centered Planning Committee: FACES (Friends and Community Experiencing Success) in MSOCS and also is a member of the State of Minnesota's Person Centered Planning Committee. She has coordinated a program called Connecting People to People within the Faribault Community and MSOCS. This program's main mission is to connect people with and without disabilities in new friendships and to foster inclusive communities. She has an associate of arts degree in liberal arts and is working on a social work degree from Mankato State University in Minnesota.

Barb Horner and the Circle Girls, Dartmouth, Nova Scotia, Canada. Barb and her husband Rich are parents of a daughter, Mallory, 19, who has multiple disabilities as a result of cerebral palsy, and a son, Josh. Mallory's friends, the Circle Girls, converge on the Horner household every 2 weeks. Mallory currently goes to high school, where she is included with her peers. Her friends have become an integral part of her life and assist her with decision making, shopping for clothes, school projects, and planning for the future. Barb and Rich continue to invite people into Mallory's life so that she will always have a strong, caring support network around her. The Horners subscribe to the idea that friends and food just naturally go together, especially when it's a group of teenagers. They believe that opportunities to connect, share life experiences, hopes, and dreams and to enjoy food together is often the foundation for life-long friendships and relationships.

Heidi Janz, Ph.D., Edmonton, Alberta, Canada, is a writer/playwright. She successfully completed her doctorate in English at the University of Alberta in April of 2003. Her dissertation, entitled *Crip Writers/Written Crips: Constructions of Illness and Disability in Selected British Poetry and Fiction*, was nominated for a Governor General's Gold Medal. Her areas of academic specialization include Disability Studies and 18th- and 19th-century poetry and fiction. She has had two plays produced: *Crips Against the Law of Gravity* and *Returned to Sender*, and recently published a novel, *Sparrows on Wheels*.

Gary McPherson, Edmonton, Alberta, Canada, has an extensive background in the voluntary sector, having spent more than 20 years in wheelchair sports administration. He served as President of the Canadian Wheelchair Sports Association. He has been inducted as a member of both the Edmonton and Alberta Sports Halls of Fame. In 1995, the University of Alberta Senate recognized his contribution to the community by awarding him an honorary doctorate of laws degree. He currently is the executive director of the Canadian Centre for Social Entrepreneurship in the School of Business at the University of Alberta. He also is an adjunct professor, as well as a special lecturer and advisor, in the faculty of Physical Education and Recreation. Prior to joining the University, Gary served for 10 years as Chairman of the Premier's Council on the Status of Persons with Disabilities, which provides advice to the Alberta Government. A biography, *Rolling On: The Story of the Amazing Gary McPherson*, from University of Alberta Press, was released in 2004. His book, *With Every Breath I Take*, is available at http://www.garymcpherson.com. In 2003, he was awarded Canada's highest honor and became a Member of the Order of Canada.

Sherrill Ruckert, Winnipeg Beach, Manitoba, Canada, has three adult children and a grandchild. She lives with her partner and works in Winnipeg at Manitoba Education and Youth, where she coordinates the production of braille for K–12 students in the province. Always interested in issues of health, Sherrill has been a tai chi instructor for many years as well as being certified in reflexology, reiki, and huna kane massage. She has studied family therapy with the Satir Professional Development Institute of Manitoba and is the Vice President of the Board for the Institute. Most recently, she is organizing a support group in Selkirk for families providing care for a family member with Alzheimer's disease under the auspices of the Alzheimer Society of Manitoba.

OTHER INVITED GUESTS

Enrico Barone and Edi Cecchini, Pisa, Italy, have two sons: Luca, 13, and Andrea, 10. The Barones are scientists, and for several years they worked in molecular genetics research. Today, they work as consultants for research groups, providing other scientists with strategies to publish and disseminate their work. Edi also manages computer courses for children and young adults with learning disabilities. Andrea has Down syndrome, and he only recently decided to begin eating solid foods. The Barones belong to the Pisa-Livorno branch of the Associazione Italiana Persone Down (AIPD). Both parents are active in the AIPD, and Enrico is the Italian Coordinator of Pedagogia dei Genitori/Parents as Educators, a section of the lifelong learning Socrates-Grudtvig2 projects of the European Union partnership. The Barones and other parents and siblings of people with disabilities want to create a European network of families, gather information on best practices in health, education, and social experiences, and groom parents and family members to become educators for other families and professionals.

Leigh Chou (a pseudonym), Coral Springs, Florida, is a stay-at-home mother/part-time computer programmer. With financial planner husband Patrick, she has two sons: Michael, 6, and Danny, 4. Danny was saying a few words by of the time he was 1, but suddenly lost all his vocabulary and didn't speak again until he was 3½. The pediatrician said to ignore it, but eventually the Chous sought other advice. Danny was diagnosed with autism and now attends a preschool for children with a variety of needs. He's beginning to speak again in complete sentences and the family is confident he'll catch up. Danny has a specific diet and doesn't tolerate gluten or dairy. The Chous are careful to explain to others that Danny's intolerance for some foods and textures is due to allergies. The Chous are also concerned that his food should be similar to that of his peers so he can be "a regular kid."

Ben Kei Daniel, Saskatoon, Saskatchewan, Canada, comes from one of the smallest tribes of the Kuku people of southern Sudan in northeastern Africa. The Kukus, mostly subsistence farmers, inhabit a small village in southwestern Sudan on the border of Uganda. The Sudan population draws from a diversity of cultures and religions, and the population speaks approximately 127 languages with 538 dialects. Household cooking and cleaning chores are not expected of people with disabilities, regardless of capability. As a result, people with disabilities contribute little and low expectations can lead to low self-worth. Ben is well versed in Sudanese cultural beliefs. He has traveled extensively and has lived in many European countries as well as Canada. He is currently a doctoral candidate doing interdisciplinary research in educational technology and computer science.

Robyn Hadfield, Armidale, Australia, is the second of five children, including a sister, Dorothy, who has Down syndrome. Robyn, a high school math teacher, lives with her husband, John, and her 7-year-old son. Two older daughters, Carmen and Emma, live away from home. Even though Robyn has lived apart from Dorothy most of her life, she says it doesn't really feel that way. Dorothy lives with her parents, who are both in their early 70s. She travels 45 kilometres from home every day to a sheltered workshop. She goes horseback riding, shopping, and to the movies on weekends and holidays. The Hadfields go to visit Dorothy and Robyn's parents at least twice a year, and Robyn's parents and Dorothy visit Robyn about once a year, with visits to the other siblings in between. Dorothy is always interested in what her siblings and her nieces and nephews are doing. Robyn wonders about her sister's future as her parents age, but says that at present, Dorothy is "quite competent, happy, and feels secure living at home with Mum and Dad."

Rod Hall, Tamworth, Australia, was born in Boggabri, Australia, in 1943, one of 11 children. His mother was a housewife and his father was a share farmer, brick maker, and school bus driver. Rod left Boggabri at 16 and went to work for Australia Post in Tamworth, where he retired 40 years later. His brother Stan, who had Down syndrome, continued to live with their parents. Rod and his wife Maxine visited on weekends and included Stan on their holidays. Stan had a stroke and died at the age of 44.

Laura Hinden, Coconut Creek, Florida, and **Rory Hoover**, Tarpon Springs, Florida, were matched in a Best Buddies friendship in 2002. Laura, 45, was born in Naples, Italy. Her father was a Navy man and she has lived in 14 different locales. In 1973, the family moved to Florida and she started high school. She started public speaking in her early 30s and recently participated in a governor's initiative for people with disabilities, and she is involved in a self-determination project with the state of Florida. Laura lives in a group home and works in a doctor's office doing clerical work.

Rory Hoover, while working at a bank in Seattle, was so inspired by an employee volunteer program that she went to Florida to attend Eckerd College in St. Petersburg, where she graduated in 2001 with a bachelor of arts degree in organizational studies for non-profits. Rory went back to work for the bank, managing the employee volunteer program for the southeast. Rory's friendship with Laura has, she says, "opened my eyes to what people with developmental disabilities can contribute and what they face every day of their lives. The physical challenges that some face are nothing compared with their isolation."

Dave Hingsburger, M.Ed., Richmond Hill, Ontario, Canada, is a speaker, author, educator, and consultant on sexuality and people with disabilities. He has provided direct care and other services for more than 25 years for people who have intellectual disabilities. He has taught in the departments of psychology and education at Bishop's University in the province of Quebec. He has written extensively, publishing books (http://www.diverse-city.com) as well as articles in newspapers, magazines, and journals. He was the focus of a documentary, *Just Say Know*, on the Discovery Channel. He wrote and produced the award-winning CBC Radio documentary *Life, Death and Disability*. Dave lectures internationally, giving keynote addresses and seminars on self-esteem for people with disabilities, abuse prevention, sexuality, sex education, and problematic sexual behavior. He is a member of the national advisory council of the Sexual Information and Education Council of Canada and is a contributing/reviewing editor for *Mental Health Aspects of Developmental Disabilities* and for the American Association on Mental Retardation journal *Mental Retardation*.

Stewart Howard (a pseudonym), Dunedoo, Australia, has a brother, Oliver (also a pseudonym), or "Ollie," who was sent to an institution when Stewart was born in 1962. The names and places related to the "Howard" family have been changed at their request due to the painful feelings associated with placing Oliver in an institution when he was a young adult. Although the names and locations are fictitious, the story is real. Like many siblings worldwide, Stewart has re-entered his brother's life in an attempt to get to know him and understand this part of his family's history.

Darlene Leister, Cudworth, Saskatchewan, Canada, lives in a shared housing unit in a rural farming community. After spending 27 years in institutions, she moved to a group home in 1988 and in 1995 moved into a more independent living arrangement. Sociable and outgoing, she is anxious to share stories about her "new life." Shelly Wiebe is a neighbor in an adjoining apartment. Both women are aided by a support worker through Columbian Industries, a vocational/residential agency.

Beth Macleod, Sydney, Australia, is a teacher. In recent years, she has developed a particular interest in students with intellectual disabilities, in part because of her own experience with her sister Margie. She recently completed a master's degree in Special Education at the University of Newcastle (New South Wales). Beth's interest in this area developed largely in response to her desire to "demystify" Margie's life and her experiences in the institution in which she lives. Margie has high support needs and was placed in the institution when she was 5 and Beth was 2. At that time, families were discouraged from having much contact with the residents, so Beth never knew her sister well. Only in recent years have they been re-establishing their bond of sisterhood. It is a process that is bringing much joy and pleasure to them both. In April 2002, Beth traveled to Canada to a week-long Planned Lifetime Advocacy Network leadership training course. She became convinced of the importance of personal relationships and networks for people with intellectual disabilities. Since then, she has been developing a friendship with Penny, another resident of the institution in which her sister lives, and is also exploring ways to strengthen Penny's personal network.

James Necula, Yorkton, Saskatchewan, Canada, and his wife **Myrna** have been married for more than 10 years. They live in a Housing Authority accessible home. Myrna uses a wheelchair and walker. The two met at a People First conference in 1988. Home Care supports Myrna with bathing, exercises, and laundry chores, and a Supportive Living Program worker helps the couple once a week. James has his own grass-cutting and snow-removal business with a fleet of equipment: a small tractor, two trailers, and a lawnmower. James declares himself the cook in the family and does most of the grocery shopping.

Kaye Pollock, Tamworth, New South Wales, Australia, teaches computing and TESOL (Teaching English to Speakers of Other Languages) in Sydney and China. She has a Teaching Diploma from Auckland Secondary Teachers' College, a bachelor of education (computer education) and a master of education (TESOL). She is the mother of three grown sons: Michael, 34; Nigel, 29; and Duncan, 26, who has spina bifida. All of her children and a grandchild reside in New Zealand. An energetic, sports-loving person, Kaye variously played and coached netball for 30 years. She lives with her husband, Gary, also an educator. When Duncan was born in Nelson, New Zealand, in 1977, doctors advised the Pollocks to institutionalize him and told them that he would likely die at age 6 months. Then at 10 months, reluctant to insert a shunt to treat hydrocephalus, one neurosurgeon pronounced that Duncan would "never be more than a cabbage." Today, Duncan has completed several Polytechnic courses in computing and community services and lives with his partner of 3 years in Hamilton, New Zealand.

Beth Porter, M.A., M.Div., is Coordinator of Educational Initiatives for L'Arche Canada, part of an international network of faith-based communities serving people with developmental disabilities. She has lived in a community of people with developmental disabilities in L'Arche for nearly 25 years. In North America, L'Arche is usually mainstream Christian in composition but is open to people of other faiths. In 1990, she began accompanying a Jewish L'Arche member who has a developmental disability to synagogue services. Beth learned how to help her prepare for her Bat Mitzvah, a celebration in which the whole L'Arche community joined. She also became committed to supporting a Muslim L'Arche member so that her faith was more recognized. This interfaith experience has been transformative for her and for her L'Arche community, which has developed a strong appreciation of what a gift it is to have people of other faiths in their midst.

Gill Rutherford, Dunedin, New Zealand, is Coordinator, Disability Studies, Dunedin College of Education. She has worked in disability/education for more than 20 years. Formerly a high school teacher, she now teaches inclusive education courses with student teachers, as well as certificate level courses with teacher aides, disability support workers, and practicing teachers. She currently is in the process of writing her doctoral dissertation, *Students with Disabilities and Teacher Aides: An Analysis of Experience.*

Robert Sanche, Saskatoon, Saskatchewan, Canada, is a retired professor, Department of Educational Psychology and Special Education, University of Saskatchewan. His teaching areas included children with disabilities in the general classroom, and transition programs and services. Robert is currently the chair of Led by the Spirit, an ecumenical group that is establishing a L'Arche community in the province.

Raffath Sayeed, Lloydminster, Alberta, Canada, is a family physician and parent of four sons, one of whom has a disability. Raffath is a former president of the Canadian Association for Community Living and is a Director of the Roeher Institute Board and the National Volunteer Organization Board. He is a former member of the Alberta Human Rights Commission and served as Acting Chief Commissioner in 1993 and 1994. His childhood in India and his work in England instilled a deep sense of appreciation for the contributions that his family has made to the history of India and to the lives of vulnerable people.

Zuhy Sayeed, Lloydminster, Alberta, Canada, has been involved in the field of differing abilities since 1982 as a parent. She has a strong background in education, having taught both in Bombay, India, and in Lloydminster. She has been involved in pressing for the inclusion of people with disabilities in a variety of capacities on the local, provincial, national, and international level. She was elected as President of the Canadian Association for Community Living in October 2003. She was appointed to the John Humphrey Centre of Peace and Human Rights, a Canadian organization working toward human rights education for children and adults.

Carl Shell, Miramar, Florida, and **Aunya Honoré,** Hallandale, Florida, had known each other for a year at the time of this book's publication. Aunya, 29, is the Citizens Program Manager of Best Buddies Florida. She met Carl, 20, when he signed up for a male Buddy. Since the two hit it off, he agreed they could spend time together "until a guy came along." Not too long afterward, Carl, who lives in a group home and works at Burger King, decided that he wanted Aunya to stay his Buddy. The pair get together a couple of times a month. They go to ball games, hockey games, bowling, dances, nature parks, and the zoo. Carl has many favorites to choose from when they go out to eat, including Chinese Buffet and Hometown Buffet restaurants. The pair attend Best Buddies functions and often just hangout by going to the movies with a meal afterwards. They keep an eye out for local events such as the Ft. Lauderdale Beach Festival, a fun time to taste various items from local restaurant vendors. Eating together, they both agree, is the time when they have their best talks. (*Note:* Just prior to publication of this book, Aunya moved to California and Carl is waiting for a new match.)

Chef Michael Smith, Fortune, Prince Edward Island, Canada, is an award-winning cookbook author, columnist, restaurant chef, mentor, and roving Canadian cuisine ambassador. He is a 1991 honors graduate of the prestigious Culinary Institute of America in New York. He has been cooking professionally for approximately 20 years. His career has included stints in a Michelin three-star restaurant in London; in some of Manhattan's finest kitchens; and in South America, the Caribbean, and throughout North America.

In 1998, Michael's first television show, *The Inn Chef,* debuted on the Life Network. *TV Guide's* readers voted it their favorite variety entertainment show on television. Michael's culinary adventure series, *Chef at Large,* debuted in 2002 and became the highest rated Canadian cooking show on Food Network Canada. Now seen in 26 countries around the world, in 2002, *Chef at Large,* won the prestigious James Beard Broadcast Media award for the best cooking show in North America. He was voted best cooking show host in Canada by the readers of the *Toronto Star*, the country's largest daily. Michael's third new series, *Chef at Home,* debuted in the fall of 2004. It features a behind-the-scenes peek at his real home kitchen and how he cooks for his family. He's currently working on his third book, also called *Chef at Home* (Whitecap, 2005).

Dick Sobsey, Ed.D., Edmonton, Alberta, Canada, began his career in human services as an attendant in a large institution, where he witnessed the abuse of people with disabilities. Over the past 25 years, he has been validating and expanding on his own experiences by working as a researcher, instructor, advocate, and consultant in the field of abuse prevention. After earning a nursing degree and a doctorate in special education, Dick started the Abuse and Disability Project at the University of Alberta, where he currently teaches in the Department of Educational Psychology. He is the director of the J.P. Das Developmental Disabilities Centre. He received the Joseph Werner American Spirit Award in 2002, and New York Governor George Pataki congratulated him on "accepting the challenge to make a difference in the lives of others." Raised in New York, Dick is the father of a son with a disability.

Roger J. Stancliffe, Ph.D., Sydney, Australia, has more than 20 years of experience working in the developmental disabilities field as a psychologist, advocate, service manager, consultant, member of the NSW Guardianship Board, researcher, and board member of non-government services. He is a consultant research associate, Research and Training Center on Community Living, Institute on Community Integration, University of Minnesota, and a Senior Research Fellow, Centre for Developmental Disability Studies, Royal Rehabilitation Centre, Sydney. He is also the editor of the *Journal of Intellectual & Developmental Disability.* His current interests include community living, deinstitutionalization, choice, self-determination, and supported open employment.

Bronwyn Thurlow, Christchurch, New Zealand, began her early childhood journey by becoming involved with her two eldest children in the setting up of a Te Kōhanga Reo, or Māori Language Nest, an indigenous early childhood movement that swept Aotearoa/New Zealand beginning in the early 1980s. Its distinguishing feature was to preserve and provide a forum for Māori language and culture. Since 1987, Bronwyn has been involved with tertiary teaching of early childhood educators, sometimes specializing in teaching introductory Māori language and tikanga (customs) to predominantly non-Māori students. She has worked in the School of Early Childhood Teacher Education/Kura Mātauranga Kaiako Kōhungahunga in the Christchurch College of Education/Te Whare Whai Mātauraka ki Ōtautahi since 1998. Bronwyn has four children. Kahurangi Marino Aroha Bronsson-George was born in 1990. He was diagnosed with Asperger syndrome at age 5.

Goomblar and Abina Wylo, Mt. Victoria, Australia. Goomblar is an Australian Aboriginal man from the Birri-Gubba and Wakka Wakka tribes of South East Queensland. He was born on the famous Aboriginal settlement Cherbourg, north of Kingaroy. Goomblar is an Aboriginal storyteller and performer who dances, sings, and plays didgeridoo (a long, hollow wooden wind instrument)—all talents passed down from elders and ancestors. He has performed on almost every continent, starred in feature films, and toured schools and universities in Australia. Goomblar and wife Abina have six children, including Murrandah, who has two very rare genetic disorders: Opitz syndrome and Kabuki syndrome. He is, says his family, the only person in the world known to have both.

Jitka Zgola, OT(C), Wreck Cove, Nova Scotia, is an occupational therapist, author, educator, and advisor to caregivers for people with Alzheimer's disease and age-related illnesses. She has more than 20 years' experience with clients, professionals, and family caregivers in direct service and administration. She provides teaching and consultation in principles of effective care to agencies and professional groups throughout Canada, the United States, and Europe, and she frequently addresses conferences as a workshop leader and keynote speaker. Early in her career, Zgola worked in pediatrics with children who had developmental disabilities, including those with spina bifida and cerebral palsy. She is the author of *Doing Things: A Guide to Activity Programming for Persons with Alzheimer's Disease* and *Care that Works: A Relationship Approach to Persons with Dementia*. With Gilbert Bordillon, international hotel/restaurant consultant, she coauthored the book *Bon Appetit! The Joy of Dining in Long-Term Care* (Health Professions Press, 2001).

Acknowledgments

He who sows courtesy reaps friendship,
and he who plants kindness gathers love.
—St. Basil

To our "family" at Paul H. Brookes Publishing Co., our appreciation in particular goes to Acquisitions Editor Rebecca Lazo for her positive and unflagging enthusiasm about this project from the beginning. To Steve Peterson, Acquisitions Assistant, we thank him for handling us gently and for his willingness to try out the recipes at home! Thanks go to Leslie Eckard, Senior Book Production Editor, for her thoughtful editing and good humor; Erin Geogheghan, Graphic Designer, for her friendly design incorporating many "ingredients," and to Amy Kopperude, Associate Production Editor, for her permissions expertise.

We also thank the Saskatchewan Association for Community Living for financial assistance for this project from both its Henderson Memorial Research Fund and the Putting Life into the Community Fund, and for the resources available through the SACL John Dolan Resource Centre. To Angela Novak Amado, Human Services Research and Development Center, St. Paul, Minnesota: Thank you for introducing us to Barb Handahl.

We thank Todd Zazelenchuk for providing an ongoing cheering section and wonderful suggestions for the reader-friendliness of the design. We are thankful to Julie Hodges for churning out all the nutritional analyses and for her good ideas to round out many of the Tidbits. Her own memories of mealtimes with her brother, who had multiple sclerosis, influence her work to develop foods for people with eating difficulties. As the MS progressed, regardless of what stage of "texture-altered" food he was eating, her brother loved the flavors and aromas and to have his family enjoying the experience of being together. Lovingly prepared food can have such power, she says, and to have family and friends be a part of mealtime experiences can enhance someone's life so much. Appreciation also goes to our pal Elizabeth Boling, whose elegant designs and drawings for the illustrated recipes and the icons give this book so much of its warm heart—and we thank her for her unflagging patience as we changed our minds more than once in mid-draw! To J. Spencer Schwier, whose brilliant folk art painting graces the cover. For his painting titled "Gathering," he took our suggestions and created a beautiful sense of family celebration and community that is the essence of this book.

Our appreciation goes to our chapter contributors for sharing their personal experiences and wisdom: Chef Michael Smith, who supplied the Foreword; to Dick Sobsey, who wrote the Introduction; and to Bill Gaventa, Barb Handahl, Barb Horner, Heidi Janz, Gary McPherson, and Sherrill Ruckert. And thanks to the following people who helped us in so many ways: Faith Bodnar, Neil Elliot, and Richard Schwier read the early manuscript and provided valuable comments and encouragement. We also thank Dr. Stephanie Baars, Los Angeles, California; Lisa Bendall, Managing Editor, *abilities*, Canadian Abilities Foundation, Toronto, Ontario; Dr. Frances Burton, University of Toronto, Ontario; Cam Crawford, The Roeher Institute, North York, Ontario; Steve Eidelman, The Arc of the United States, Silver Spring, Maryland; Richard Gehring, Buffalo & Erie County Meals on Wheels, Buffalo, New York; Shirley Gerein, administrator, Biggar Group Home, Biggar, Saskatchewan; Karen Green McGowan, McGowan Consultants, Georgia; Dana Guernsey, Herkimer Area Resource Center, Peachtree City, New York; Shelley Hourston, B.C. Coalition of People with Disabilities, Vancouver, British Columbia; Dave Hingsburger, Diverse City Press, Richmond Hill, Ontario; June Isaacson Kailes, Disability Policy Consultant, Western University of Health Sciences, Pomona, California; Gill Rutherford, College of Education, Dunedin, New Zealand; James Schwier, Whisky's, Lawrenceburg, Indiana; Hazel Self, Gage Transition to Independent Living, Toronto, Ontario; Roger Stancliffe, Royal Rehabilitation Centre, Sydney, Australia; Nancy Wallace-Gero, Community Living Essex County, Ontario; Chef Dave White, Cincinnati, Ohio; Larry Youse, Grand Finale, Cincinnati, Ohio; Dr. Jitka Zgola, Giverny Consultants, Wreck Cove, Nova Scotia; and probably several more we regrettably but undoubtedly have missed.

Particular thanks go to all of the individuals and families in the United States, Canada, New Zealand, Sudan, Ireland, Italy, and Australia whose stories and observations are the "soul food" of this project.

Foreword

An Appetizer

As a professional chef, I have learned many things about cooking and food, but no lesson has been more powerful than what I learned as a small boy at the dining room table. Surrounded on a daily basis by loving family and colorful friends, I discovered that food at its best is meant to be shared with others, to feed not only the body but also the soul.

I have been blessed with a long and productive career. I have cooked for kings, queens, presidents, and Hollywood celebrities. I have scaled mountains, pushed through wilderness, rode out storms, and found my way home. While I'm proud of my professional accomplishments, none compare to the simple joy of cooking a meal for friends and family.

While some of us take breaking bread for granted, many of us anticipate and savor the experience. In particular for people with disabilities, it's a time to share life with others. The simple act of preparing and eating food together reinforces the humanity in us all. There are no limitations at my table.

When life is partly defined by what you can't do, the simple ceremonies of a meal take on added significance. The table is a place of equals where all who sit down bring a part of themselves to share with others and, in turn, enrich themselves. This interchange has been part of civilization since free-range dinosaurs last appeared on menus! It's part of what makes us human.

The fundamental human need to share a meal with others presents a powerful opportunity to enhance the sense of belonging and community in a life that often craves such normalcy. Simple interaction with others reaffirms humanity. It's not just about food; it's about being yourself and letting go of life's restrictions. It's the joy of the table. *Breaking Bread, Nourishing Connections* is much like a good cookbook in the hands of a thoughtful, caring chef. Preparing food, cooking, and sharing it with others is so much more than just reading off a list of ingredients. A good chef does much more than just assemble and combine. A good chef chooses a cookbook that has heart and passion, one that compels the reader to try new things and share that with family and friends. A good cookbook gives you a sense of the celebration, the welcome, the involvement that is a joyful mealtime. A good chef understands that the food may be what draws us together, but what makes us come back for more is the human interaction and joyful celebration we create at table. This book reminds us what is important and why. That is the contribution I think *Breaking Bread, Nourishing Connections* will make.

Chef Michael Smith
Chef at Home
Chef at Large
Food Network Canda

Introduction

Searching for Sustenance

Back in the 1980s, I begged Paul H. Brookes Publishing Co. to let me write a book called *Mealtime Skills for People with Severe and Multiple Disabilities*. When I finally got the green light, I was raring to go. In fact, I even had a pretty good head start.

I had completed my doctoral dissertation on eating and feeding skills a few years earlier, complete with the customary comprehensive review of the literature. After that, I published some articles on nutrition and food textures, and I had written a pretty comprehensive chapter on mealtime skills for a text that was generally well received. In fact, when I thought about it carefully, food and mealtimes had been prominent in my writing from the very beginning of my career. The very first piece that I ever sold as a writer was "Getting Started with Maple Syrup." I still display the $50 check stub from Rodale Press in my office with great pride, even though it is clearly marked "to be used as filler in coming issue of *Organic Gardening and Farming*." Any way that I looked at it, I was ready.

When I sat down in front of the blank computer screen to write, however, I did not feel ready. I had the distinct feeling that something important was left out of the equation. I knew that some other voice needed to be heard. I sensed that something had changed. It took a long time to figure out what that was, but now it seems obvious.

What was missing from the book was its soul. I will not try to convince you that all books have souls, but I have certainly convinced myself that good ones do. A book's soul is simply an emotional spark that gives a book life, something that runs under the words, that speaks to the reader's heart. Without it, authors can fill pages with information, but they cannot breathe life into them.

The missing voice had only just begun to speak to me. Like a song carried on the wind, the voice was so soft back then that I could not make out all the words and yet the melody was compelling. It was the voice of my own son, David, and a chorus of others who, like him, have severe disabilities. Even today, I am not quite sure that I have gotten the message exactly right. But it goes something like this: *Give us food, but also give us sustenance. Feed our bodies, but also nourish us with the stuff of life. Share with us the fruit of the vine and wheat that springs from the earth, but also join us in a celebration of the human spirit.*

The thing that had changed was me. In between writing the prospectus for my text and actually writing the book, our son David was born with severe and multiple disabilities and I was transformed. When I say that I was transformed, I mean that it changed the way that I look at the world and the universe. Even now, 13 years later, I am still learning and changing. Nevertheless, even at the earliest stages of my metamorphosis, it was clear to me that the book that I had envisioned writing was no longer relevant. Unfortunately, I was not far along enough in the change process to envision a better one. Yet, as the years went on, some of the necessary revisions became clear to me. For example, the old book would have a chapter on nutrition that would tell people to ensure adequate vitamin D intake and avoid sugary foods with empty calories that rot the teeth. The new book would have a section on sustenance for the heart that would have its own list of essential foods. *Every child should eat birthday cake regularly at the parties of real friends.* If the book that I originally had envisioned was about *Mealtime Skills,* the book that I began to envision was more like *Dinner with David.*

This is not to say that there is no place for technical information in a book about mealtimes. On the contrary, technical information is essential, but it is insufficient without the human dimension of mealtimes. The ideal book has both.

I never got around to writing that book; however, in many ways, Karin Melberg Schwier and Erin Schwier Stewart have written the book I envisioned—a blend of practical information on eating and feeding with the heart and soul of mealtimes. They've prepared a feast and invited some great guests, and I am delighted to join them at the table. Looking at the guest list, I see the names of some old friends and the names of some interesting new acquaintances. Each guest has brought a contribution of his or her own creation to the celebration. The menu looks enticing, and there is plenty to go around. So, on behalf of everyone involved, I invite you the reader to join us and dig in!

Dick Sobsey, Ed.D.
Director,
J.P. Das Developmental Disabilities Centre
University of Alberta, Canada

JUST FOR STARTERS

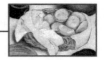

CHAPTER 1

Food for Thought

Mealtime is a spacer.
It's such a nice way to travel
Between each of the other moments in life.
It's a breath between getting from and going to,
And at the same time, it's somewhere to be.
—MARC AND RONNA GOLD (AS CITED IN PERSKE, CLIFTON, MCLEAN, & STEIN, 1986)

Food.

We hunt, catch, gather, grow. We prepare it, present it, share it, and show it off. Babies howl for it. Cruise ship chefs fashion it into elaborate statues that look too good to eat. Hunters chase down their dinner on the savannah, and gatherers pluck it out from under rocks in the sea.

Food is often the very foundation of religious faith and fellowship; it is the embodiment of Spirit. A Thai friend says the standard greeting in her family isn't "How are you?" but rather "Have you eaten yet?" Newlyweds share pieces of their wedding cake for good luck, to the delight of family and friends. We tend our gardens and share the bounty with our neighbors. In every culture of the world, food represents a focal point of human interaction, celebration, and ceremony.

Food consumes us. During all stages of life, from birth through death, we eat, and when we are not eating, we are thinking about food. Those of us who are lucky have it every single day of our lives; those who don't, suffer. Food and all its attendant activities and rituals make various cultures unique, yet link us all by a common need. Food influences family and community responsibilities and roles. Adults organize their lives around mealtimes, and children learn about taking turns and sharing through food-related activities. Recreation and leisure pursuits involve cooking and eating. We boast about going to cooking schools in Santa Fe and Tuscany, and we regale friends with stories about vacations based on where we ate what, sometimes complete with photos of the food partaken. We read food magazines and watch cooking shows. People take food preparation, fast-food, and dishwashing jobs during school and have careers as cod fishers, farmers, or gourmet chefs.

When you think about it, mealtime is a renewable resource of opportunity for people to spend time together. It is a reason for people to gather together in a way that is uniquely human. This gathering to share food seems to know no boundaries of race, culture, religion, age, or ability level. It can be a great social equalizer for people with and without disabilities. It can simply be an excuse to come together and enjoy one another's company in a way that does not focus on strengths or needs, program plans, or assessments. It's just a wonderfully simple, everyday reason to be together. As grandparents in every culture for generations have insisted, "You gotta eat!"

A MOTIVATING FORCE

If mealtime is a renewable resource, then food is a social lubricant that can keep the machinery of involvement and interaction running between people with and without disabilities. Many families, personal network members, friends, advocates, and service providers who interact most closely each day with individuals who have disabilities see the value of mealtimes and kitchen tasks in promoting emotional and physical well-being.

Merely consuming food at the expense of doing other activities is, of course, not what we're talking about. Far too many people with disabilities have had a disservice done to them by well-meaning family and caregivers. One might hear such people say, "He just loves to eat. And it's the only thing he's interested in, so why not keep him happy?" Well, he could have a heart attack, for one thing! This type of caring can lead to obesity and its associated health risks. Individuals with disabilities also may lack informed choices or opportunities to engage in a range of other activities.

This book looks at food and all of the activities associated with it as a motivating force to energize and activate relationships between people with and without disabilities and within families and communities. Often, families and human services providers search for inclusive social activities. Meals and mealtimes lend themselves easily to such inclusive gatherings and are so readily available; they present themselves at least two or three times every day literally right under our noses.

Families and service providers sometimes arrange for the individuals they serve to have meals out, and some agencies have cooking programs for the people who live within those services. Supper clubs and lunch groups also provide individuals with ways to socialize and learn cooking skills. Often, however, these types of activities tend to be restricted to the people who live within the agency, so opportunities for individuals with and without disabilities to form new relationships and learn new skills do not always exist. Says Steve Eidelman, Executive Director of The Arc of the United States:

> *In some places, meal preparation is still seen as staff work, for all the wrong reasons. In still others—especially the ICFMR (Intermediate Care Facility—Mental Retardation program)—if it's not in someone's plan, then it does not happen.*

Some agencies, regrettably, seem paralyzed by liability fears, and they create policies that prevent people with disabilities from being in the kitchen where they might alternatively 1) burn, 2) cut, or 3) scald themselves, or the ever-popular 4) make a mess. Eidelman agrees, and he lists a variety of other reasons for why the kitchen is seen as out of bounds for some people with disabilities:

> *In yet other agencies, the job of food preparation and clean up is kept from people with disabilities because it takes too long. It is viewed as inefficient. It is messy and there is the ever-present fear of liability. All lame excuses depriving people of one of life's great pleasures.*

Life skills and community access programs for people with disabilities often include field trips to the grocery store. Sometimes, these experiences may be useful to individuals. Sometimes, however, these outings are not so productive. The people with disabilities end up floating along after the shopping cart like so many dinghies "tied" to the staff person, who makes all of the selections and steers the course. We have a friend with a disability who is 45. He has a full-time job. He's never learned to cook, and every day he takes a lunch to work that a staff person makes for him. It's always the same: an uninteresting sandwich on white bread, a couple of carrots sticks, a cookie wrapped nicely in plastic wrap, and a juice box—a lunch that would make a fifth grader happy.

We're suggesting that all of the tasks associated with mealtime—such as making one's own lunch and trying new foods—can be prime opportunities for an individual to join other people and revel in their company, learn new skills, show off abilities, and be a grown-up. Hopefully, agencies and designers of human services are becoming more enlightened about the value of mealtimes and a sense of home for the people they serve. You'll find great examples in this book of some ways service providers are making their services feel less institutional and more like those you would find at your home.

Although some agencies put great effort into volunteer programs that match people with and without disabilities, largely through group activities but also in "buddy" pairings and one-to-one activities, most of the activities do not involve mealtimes. Sure, a once-a-month trip to a fast-food restaurant is a fun outing. But it shouldn't be the only mealtime experience, particularly if there is no real participation or involvement in the outing other than consuming a giant hamburger.

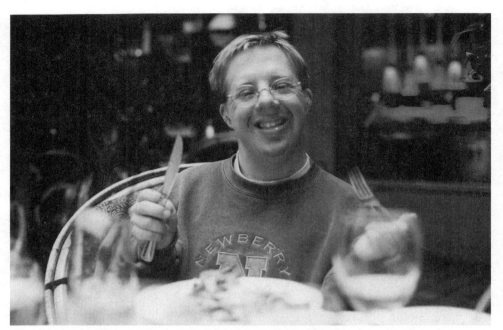

Knowing which fork to use first and handling oneself well during dinner conversation can boost anyone's self-esteem.

Mealtime should be a much more interactive human activity. We are members of complex families, so we're not so naïve as to think that every mealtime is going to be a relaxed, open opportunity for people to sit around the table, giving and receiving emotional sustenance as well as sharing good food. Sometimes people are in a hurry. Sometimes a drive-through meal is necessary to keep on schedule. Sometimes people aren't in the best of moods or there's a crisis in progress that puts a damper on mealtime connections. But if we pause for a moment and remind ourselves about the possibilities for connections inherent in mealtime activities, we have a goal to work toward.

WHAT IS MEALTIME?

So what do we mean by *mealtime* for the purposes of this book? As authors intimately connected to family and friends with disabilities, we propose an expanded definition. We are looking at mealtime opportunities for people of all ages, cultures, and living situations; for people with friends and without; and for people whose disabilities are profoundly challenging as well as for those who can, with a little support, participate easily. To us, no disability precludes the sharing of an enjoyable mealtime experience. These opportunities for intimate, one-to-one interactions we collectively call mealtime—including planning, shopping, selecting, preparing, and eating—can involve all sorts of skills, talents, information gathering, community presence, social value, sensory experiences, and human involvement.

Think of all of the jobs involved, for example, in a simple dinner gathering for a few friends. A lovely presentation of Singapore noodles doesn't magically appear on the table—even though there are days we wish it would. All of the tasks that go into the meal begin well before the food is placed on the table, and they continue well after the last person lays down a fork with a satisfied smacking of lips (or, depending on the culture, other sounds that may be appropriate indicators of enjoyment!).

Just think of all of the tasks involved in one dinner party (whether it is for a special occasion or just a casual get-together):

- Planning the meal
- Inviting guests
- Accommodating the likes and needs of the guests
- Choosing the menu
- Hunting down the ingredients
- Purchasing the ingredients
- Getting ready in the kitchen
- Dressing for the occasion
- Cooking
- Assembling the dishes
- Cleaning the house
- Setting the table
- Lighting candles and arranging flowers
- Choosing the music
- Welcoming guests
- Making people feel comfortable
- Offering appetizers and drink
- Sharing each other's company at the table
- Serving the meal
- Eating the meal
- Putting on the coffee or tea
- Offering dessert
- Serving the dessert
- Clearing away
- Washing up
- Remembering to relax
- Enjoying the company of friends

That's a lot of activity! Each of these activities has dozens of associated tasks that can be shared in a meaningful way to ensure that a family member or friend with a disability can feel uplifted, enthused, and energized.

Why This Book?

The very fact that you are reading this book means that you have already thought about how you might become involved in the life of someone with a disability, or you would like to introduce new experiences and a deeper commitment to the relationships you already have. We think mealtime is an excellent opportunity to do that.

We hope this book will become a valuable resource for family members, friends, next-door neighbors, potential community connections, members of wider support networks, and residential services staff who experience mealtimes every day with people who have disabilities.

This book provides some ideas, strategies, and suggestions that may be helpful as you get to know someone better and spend more time together and as you think through how you might make your interactions more comfortable. We also hope to put your mind at ease about sharing mealtimes with an individual or people with disabilities who may need extra support to participate. Many types of utensils, cups, plates, bowls, and kitchen gadgets are available to make cooking and eating easier for people with and without disabilities. There are also ways of sitting and positioning for people who have too much or too little muscle tone, for example, which help with the dining experience. Distractions can be minimized, as well. Strategies can be implemented to ensure that a person with a disability enjoys choice making and control and places your time together on an equal footing. We also offer some ideas for you to consider about someone with a disability and her[1] contribution to a relationship and the wider community.

Tidbits

Throughout this book and gathered together in Appendix B, you will come across tidbits of information and ideas that you may find helpful depending on the person with whom you are spending mealtimes. Watch for these tidbits, which are categorized in this manner:

Safety and Health

These tidbits offer advice on creating experiences that are safe for everyone involved, which provide the dignity of risk and promote healthy choices and activities.

---

[1]To be fair to both genders in describing individuals in this book, pronouns will be alternated.

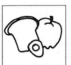

Good Idea

Sometimes the best ideas for ways to connect and interact with people are the simplest ones. We provide a selection of ideas gathered from families, friends, and service providers as well as from people with disabilities. This collection offers various ideas that will make you say, "Why didn't I think of that?"

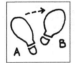

Food for Thought

Providing support to people with disabilities in a way that promotes equality can be sharpened by reflection. A variety of these tidbits will provide an opportunity to consider your own beliefs, values, and role perceptions of people with disabilities and how a change in attitude and practice can occur.

Positioning

Usually you don't need to be specially trained to assist someone who needs some adaptations or physical support to participate in mealtime. But you can learn much from the person himself or his family and caregivers. We offer some ways to make the person comfortable and at ease during mealtimes.

Gadgets

Small adaptations to common utensils and/or different designs of items used for a variety of mealtime tasks can make a big difference in someone's comfort and independence. Offered are a variety of suggestions for adapting what you already have and sources for new items that make life easier.

Stories

As authors, many of our perspectives come from experiences with our own family and friends and, in particular, our son/brother Jim who has an intellectual disability. But you'll also find stories throughout this book from people with disabilities and family members and friends. You can "meet" these individuals in About the Contributors starting on page xi. We like to think of these personal stories as sprinkles: colorful slices of personal perspectives, advice, suggestions, and experiences to help us understand the vast array of mealtime meanings.

Activities

Chapter 2 includes activities to help you understand the issues related to mealtimes and how to make them more fun, comfortable, and dignified for both you and your dinner companions. These are easy to practice and implement.

Recipes

We offer a number of recipes in Appendix A, many of which have been illustrated and adapted to use plain language. They have been tested from start to finish by professionals in the field of nutrition and by people with disabilities and their friends, family, and staff. Share these recipes, and also use the recipe template to tailor your own favorites. We encourage people to spend fun time in the kitchen together, creating something impressive to show off.

What This Book Is Not

This book is not a step-by-step "how to" that will show you what to say and do and when in every occasion. The fact is that people with disabilities may have different ways to communicate; mealtimes can be a time when you naturally build on that. People have different physical needs and not everybody is going to be able to twirl spaghetti with ease. By spending time together, we learn each other's likes and dislikes, our strengths and our needs. We figure out together how to be together. We begin with the belief that sharing mealtimes is a positive, enriching experience. The practical ideas, adaptations, and techniques developed by families and professionals such as occupational therapists break down barriers and flow from that inclusive belief.

The American Occupational Therapy Association (AOTA) has stated that, "Occupational therapy supports and encourages the ordinary and familiar things that people do every day" (1995, p. 1015) that bring purpose, meaning, enjoyment, and satisfaction into their lives. This simple idea may be especially inviting for a companion or volunteer who would like to spend time with someone who has a disability, but who isn't sure how to break the experience into smaller tasks or who needs to help in learning to meet the individual's needs. This is not an occupational therapy textbook, although one of the authors has practical experience and expertise as an occupational

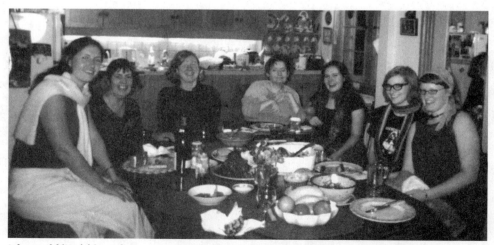

A feast of friendship welcomes an English relative, several old and new friends and past and current care providers to the Schaefer house in Winnipeg, Canada, a gathering that pleases Catherine, center.

therapist in educational and medical settings and provides helpful suggestions to aid readers in developing relationships. It is not our intention to "therapize" mealtimes. In fact, the last thing we want to do is scare off connections for people with disabilities by implying that a potential friend or neighbor requires occupational therapy training in order to make a batch of biscuits together. We're talking about how to make mealtimes pleasurable and enjoyable for everybody involved.

Tips for Getting to Know Someone

Probably the best advice we can give is to *get to know the person*. Use this list of questions as a guide for conducting your "research" about who this person is and how you might help him understand who you are. Both partners in the interaction should answer these questions, if possible; they are not only for people with disabilities. When you think about it, very few of these questions have to do with disability:

- What does an ordinary day look like? Do I plan the things I will do?
- Am I happy with my days?
- Are there days in my week that I like more than others? Why?
- Who are the people I know?
- Who are my friends? How did I meet them? Do I have a boyfriend or girlfriend?
- What do I do with my friends?
- What do I have in common with my friends?
- Who is paid to be in my life?
- What are my relationships with others like?
- What is my best characteristic?
- What things do I own?
- What do I do for fun?
- What are my favorite things to do?
- What are my hobbies?
- Who can I talk to about private things? Can I trust this person?
- What kind of physical contact do I have in my life? Is it my choice? Who loves me?
- How do I communicate? How do I make others know what I want?
- What makes me sad?
- What makes me happy?
- What do I do for work? Do I enjoy it? Do I get paid, or do I volunteer?
- What am I proud of?
- What things do I have some say over and choices about? How do I express my choices?

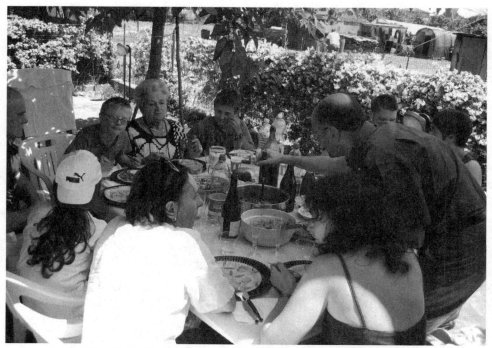

In a Pisa backyard, Enrico ladels out the Zuppa Toscana during a mealtime that lasts several hours. One does not rush a meal in Italy. *Noi non mangiarmo per vivere, viviamo per mangiare.* (One does not eat to live, one lives to eat.)

Sometimes it takes time to establish a comfortable rapport with someone who has a disability. By focusing on common elements of humanity, you can sidestep the tricky quicksand of disability and merely think of each other as potential friends. Mealtime is a valuable commodity; small moments traded from time to time can nourish lasting connections.

HAVING THE TIME OF OUR LIVES

The other and equally important meaning of mealtime is that of attention and participation. Whether people with and without disabilities are together for a dinner at home or a picnic in the park, the critical ingredient is that each person is devoted to the others for that time. What is it about mealtimes that allow people to pay attention to one another?

In a world geared to "faster" and "more," we're driven to continually juggle several tasks in our race to eventually clear our to-do lists so that we'll have that elusive thing called *time*. Pat Katz is a Canadian speaker and writer who helps people make the most of the time in their lives. The author of the e-zine, *PAUSE: The Voice of Sanity in a Speed Crazed World* [http://www.patkatz.com], reminds people to "give yourself permission to pause." In a world of indiscriminate multitasking, she fears relationships are too often put on hold as the clock and the weight of daily expectations drive people to distraction. But mealtime, she says, can help us to slow down:

> *You can peel potatoes or wash dishes and have a wonderful conversation. However, you can't fully attend to a conversation while checking your e-mail, listening to phone messages, and catching the news on television. What makes mealtimes magic? It's because the other appliances and distractions of our lives are set aside, turned off, or ignored.*

Katz is an advocate of no television, radio, computers, or telephone calls (and that includes text messaging!) during a meal:

> *At mealtime, we are gathered around a table, face to face, eye to eye. It's that same kind of opportunity for attention—this time supplemented by the caring preparation and service of good food. It's another form of nourishment.*

Ultimately, aside from all of the focus on the food itself, mealtime is this: a break to relax, time to talk, time to laugh, a respite from technological distractions, a chance to savor with our senses, and a time to notice and nourish one another.

Mealtime doesn't look the same in every culture or in every family or household. An occasional TV dinner shared in front of *Wheel of Fortune*, samosas and hammer sauce at the farmer's market, hot dogs and Cokes at the Reds game, or an elaborate Kwanzaa feast with far-flung relatives and every trimming all provide rich opportunities for sharing and companionship.

Such Richness

Eating together is, or can be, such a rich time for interaction. If someone needs some assistance to shower or dress, for instance, the time spent with that person doing that activity is relatively short. But mealtime is longer and more sociable with other people. In the residential unit at the institution where Margie lives, this sort of interaction doesn't often happen. There are about four staff scheduled there at a time, and there are 22 residents. So they just don't have time to sit down and spend 15 minutes with each person during a meal. But when we take her out, we interact with her a lot. Also, when we go out for ice cream with chocolate sauce, her favorite, she loves to watch people. Sometimes she eats fast, and I think that is probably a result of institutional living. Whatever is put in front of you is yours and you take it and don't let anyone else get it! But when we go out, she often puts her spoon down to watch people going by. It's lovely to see her enjoying the activity going on around her. When Margie comes to our home, mealtimes have something of a celebratory feel. I guess there's a tactile aspect to it, too, as we are touching as I assist her. Mealtime often feels like a rich time. I'm not good at analyzing it. We're just doing something we both enjoy, eating and drinking! It's a mutual pleasure. —Beth Macleod, Australia

Recipe Box Letter #5

Grandma's lemon pie
the last piece halved
between my brother and me
and up to me to
cut or choose.

Dead-eye down the middle
a steady hand makes
two from one

my brother's little nose
poised a hair above the plate
weighing the smell of each slice
until nothing is held in the balance
those quivering wedges sparking
the blue right out of his eyes
with food-lust.

Pie can stretch a night out.
Mom's fuming for bath and bed
but she can't touch us—

eat the meringue
wave by wave, brown ones last,
let the bubbled surface melt
onto my tongue,
lick the flakes of crust
one at a time
from the back of my fork
swirl each bite of filling
inside my mouth
until it runs down my
satisfied throat.

Shout to my brother
his must have been smaller
'cuz he finished first
as Mom hoists him by the elbow
over the running tub.

We still meet sometimes
in sleep
carving out a world of pie
past our bedtimes.
—MICHAEL BRADFORD (2004)

"Recipe Box #5" by Michael Bradford, from the book *Personal Effects*, published by Coteau Books. Used by permission of the publisher.

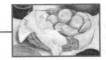

CHAPTER 2

Feeding or Dining?

Some children like to make castles out of rice pudding,
or faces with raisins for eyes . . . Let's all play with our food,
I say, and, in so doing, let us advance the state of the art together.
—JULIA CHILD (FROM THE SWIVEL COLLECTIVE, 2002)

Intellectually, we understand that *feeding* implies the physical input of nutrition. Technically, feeding means putting food in someone's mouth—or introducing nutrition in some manner. Family members and people with disabilities fear, however, that the term has been bastardized to the point that it implies a chore, part of the caregiver's job (and a messy one at that). Although many people use this term in a benign way, it's important to appreciate the climate in which many people with disabilities live. This "the residents have to be fed" attitude, in our view, strips people with disabilities of competence and dignity; it is one more thing *done to* them rather than *done with* them.

THE DEEPER MEANING OF DINING

Dining, in contrast, has deeper contextual meaning. Dining implies something beyond the physical act of getting food into oneself or someone else. Dining suggests something more transcendent and, without making it too grandiose, maybe even something more spiritual. Can standing over the sink shoulder-to-shoulder with a family member or a friend, polishing off a big pan of brownies together, be a dining experience? We think so!

What makes up an enjoyable dining experience? Can it be put into words or given a strict definition agreed on by all? As a comparison, ask yourself this: How do

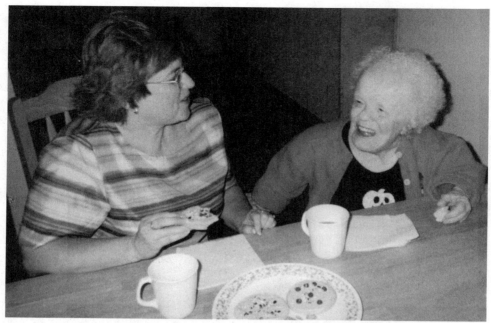

Food is usually part of Michelle (left) and Ethel's time together. Michelle has known Ethel for more than 25 years, first as a high school student volunteer, and now as Ethel's conservator (a type of guardian). When the institution in Minnesota in which Ethel lived was closing, Michelle advocated for Ethel to stay near her because Ethel had no family in her home county.

we know if we are loved? How can we be sure we are loved and that someone isn't just going through the motions? Perhaps we don't really know unless we have experienced it. "Touch and talk, coo and stroke, murmur and caress—the very first lessons children need to learn is that they are valuable and desirable beings" (Melberg Schwier, & Hingsburger, 2000, p. 25). Without those early, intangible lessons in safety and security, we may grow up feeling that perhaps there is something wanting in us, something lacking, a disturbing feeling that is never pinpointed. We think the difference between being fed and sharing a meal, or *dining,* is just as fundamental.

Dining more aptly describes the meaning, activities, and context of consuming food. It suggests a shared activity rather than an act someone does to another person. Dining does not necessarily mean nibbling expensive shrimp scampi on Noritake china with gleaming Reed and Barton silver. Rather, it is a more interactive, organic experience that goes beyond—sometimes above and beyond—giving and receiving nutrition. Larry Youse is an award-winning Cincinnati restaurateur. He has graced the cover of *Bon Appétit* magazine. His star-studded restaurant, Grand Finale, established in 1975, has won numerous awards including the *Cincinnati Magazine's* Hall of Fame for 10 years running and the Mobil Three Stars award for 20 years. When he's asked to describe what he strives for at his establishment, he responds "Consistent good taste." Then he adds:

But let me be more specific. Consistent good taste means the experience from the moment you enter our property to the moment you leave. That includes the condition of our building and landscaping, ease of entrance, smiling faces, beautiful interiors, clean restrooms and dining rooms, an immaculate kitchen, friendly and competent service, quiet and well-mannered bussers, charming hostesses in complete control, and then, to top that off, food that tastes good and food that is a good value. When I say consistent good taste, I mean only a portion is what you taste with your taste buds. Equally as important is what you taste with your eyes and ears.

Still, we may not fully appreciate the significant difference between feeding and dining if we have not had the chance to compare the two. One of the easiest ways to do this is to make some stark comparisons between historical practices and what we strive for today.

A Historical Perspective

In 1977, a book by Perske, Clifton, McLean, and Stein exploded across a collective consciousness in the United States. *Mealtimes for Severely and Profoundly Handicapped Persons* grew out of a Random House study commissioned by the federal government's Health, Education and Welfare Office. The original intent was to seek out and offer up cutting-edge practices in a variety of services for people with severe and profound disabilities. Robert Perske, noted advocate and award-winning author, led the team, and over the course of a year, the study took an interesting shift.

Surprisingly, concerns about mealtime kept rising to the surface. Comments about how "We'd better start doing it [helping people eat] right" and "There must be a better way" in terms of mealtimes for people with disabilities kept popping up between the information about great therapy programs and other institutional management practices. Perske and his team soon realized that the focus of this study had to be a recognition of mealtime as an important aspect in the lives of people living in institutions. Karen Green McGowan is a registered nurse with advanced certification in developmental disabilities nursing. She manages a Georgia-based consulting firm specializing in training, evaluation, publications, and technical assistance to organizations serving individuals with complex developmental disabilities, intellectual disabilities, cerebral palsy, and challenging health problems. Green McGowan is one of the originators of the person-centered planning process. She worked in wards for people with disabilities in the mid-1960s and early 1970s. She remembers many deaths; too many were food-related. In an era in which death rates were high in residential settings for people with severe disabilities, too many people choked on food. Paraphrasing from *Implementing Person-Centered Planning: Voices of Experience* (2002), Green McGowan reflects on research "replete with data that suggests for the most physically challenged, aspiration pneumonia is a major cause of death." She adds:

Aspiration was the major cause of death for most people with neuro-developmental problems and continues to be so to this day, although the rates are much lower because of better seating, positioning, and therapeutic approach technology.

In the state facility in which I worked, there were initially two to three deaths a month in a facility of 1,200. Most of these deaths were directly related to swallowing issues. Of course, in those days, we had no positioning equipment, and so a lot of folks got fed lying flat on their backs during the 60 minutes that two staff were allotted to help 30 totally dependent people eat. Needless to say, aspiration is still the major cause of death in children and adults with complex neuromotor disabilities.

Perske, Green McGowan, and many others were hearing too many disturbing stories to ignore them. Robert Perske notes:

One that really shook us was in North Carolina at Morganton. Some people came up with this really simple time–motion study. The minute the food cart would go into a ward, on their stopwatches would go. When the food cart came out, they stopped their watches. All they had to do was count the number of people who had their mealtime—they called it "feeding"—and our team decided to never call it that—and they computed an average of 4.8 minutes per person. Just think. I remember working in the institutions where we did a lot of "bird feeding" and we kind of dreamed a lot about why couldn't people have a nice meal with some ambiance to it. You know, the kind where people sit around the table and really do break bread. People share things; here, have a little of this. Try some of that. People laugh and it's a beautiful time together.

Why couldn't it be like this for people with disabilities? Perske dreamed of pleasant mealtimes for people with disabilities that would last longer than 4.8 minutes. In the book's introduction, he regretfully described what many people believed to be best practices of the day. Even as professionals struggled to create some sense of normalcy in large institutions, it was virtually impossible to normalize the living conditions of thousands of people, many of whom had complex needs. Parents were frustrated, exhausted, and ill informed about how best to support sons and daughters with serious disabilities who still lived at home. But even those caregivers who were supposed to provide professional care were not always making the lives of people with disabilities pleasant, secure, or even safe.

Families and professionals of the day voiced relief when these archaic practices began to fade as people started to realize how insensitive and downright dangerous they were. We dare say the way it was is pretty far removed from an evening at the Grand Finale. This list of what one nurse called "quiet little murders" (Perske et al., 1986, p. xix) is the reason, Perske says, a gentle call was mounted to revolutionize the practices that robbed people of not only their dignity and humanity but also their health—

and occasionally—their lives. These practices, Perske wrote (Perske et al. 1986), included the following:

- *Tube-feeding*: People who have had a gastrostomy must eat through a plastic tube that is placed into a surgically prepared orifice in their stomachs. Food passes into the stomach through the tube. Although tube-feeding may be necessary in acute situations, in some situations or organizations it has been ordered because it is perceived to save costs or staff time. "Fortunately," Perske says, "we now recognize how psychologically devastating this kind of experience can be when it is used unnecessarily."

- *Bird feeding*: This is the practice, no longer used much today, of holding a person's chin up and to pour food down his throat; people prided themselves on being able to do this without spilling. This kind of feeding often resulted in food going into the lungs instead of down to the stomach, which was determined to be a factor in deaths due to aspiration pneumonia. Most caregivers today are aware of the dangers associated with this.

- *Rapid feeding*: Administrators in some institutions and organizations became concerned with the practice of rapid mealtimes—in one case the superintendent and other staff discovered that less than 5 minutes was spent per person. This kind of inhumane rapid feeding led to the reorganization of staffing patterns so that people could have more leisurely mealtimes.

- *Feeding on the back*: Leaving people to lie on their backs while being fed was at one time considered less work and less mess. Luckily, people realized that eating while lying down on one's back feels terrible, and similar to bird-feeding, can cause aspiration pneumonia. "Today, many service training programs have simulated sessions where caregivers are fed on their backs. Once they know how it feels, they understand why it is important to avoid using this position unless they have to," Perske notes.

- *Undesirable atmospheres*: Some dining rooms in institutions and group homes have very noxious atmospheres, unpleasant smells, and chaotic movement of residents and staff. "Regimented eating in Oliver Twist dining halls may be tolerable on rare occasions, but a steady three-times-a-day experience can easily contribute to maladaptive behaviors and psychological retreat," Perske adds.

- *Puréed food*: Some people need food in puréed or liquid forms, but anyone who has ever tasted baby food should know that whenever possible, a goal should be to plan for the day when a person on a puréed diet will be able to graduate to more solid foods that are more tasteful and offer a wider range of nutrients. Many people with disabilities are able to do this in a planned program supervised by a physician.

- *Insensitivity to reachable developmental goals*: In the past, no thought was given to how mealtimes provide rich opportunities for sensory development; social and emotional growth; and the development of self-help, fine and gross motor, and decision-making skills. Fortunately, people are now realizing the potential of meal-times for all kinds of growth.

As of the publication of *Breaking Bread, Nourishing Connections,* more than 25 years had passed since Perske's *Mealtimes* was first released. The impact of those insti-tutional practices still lingers, however. Although many people moved back into more home-like settings in the community, sometimes the idea that people require institu-tional treatment has followed them to their new homes. As family members, we worry that a new generation of human service workers may miss out on the lessons Perske and his team came to appreciate. Despite current thinking about what people with disabilities are capable of in terms of enjoying mealtimes, some may still wonder, "What's the big deal about being fed versus dining?" We are conscious of stories told by people with disabilities themselves.

Pete Park is a Canadian who spent 18 years living at the Oxford Regional Centre near Woodstock, Ontario. The food, he recalls, was "less than interesting" for the hun-dreds of residents with TB, epilepsy, and intellectual disabilities.

> Regularly, everybody got oatmeal with, oh, I don't know, coulda been yesterday's breakfast in it. Anything they could steam boil, they steam boil. Steamed food. Cripes! Until you couldn't even tell if it was a vegetable. You could sorta tell if it was green or orange, but that was about it. On Fridays, we always had fish so we nicknamed it Fish Friday. Steamed fish. You could smell the cotton pickin' stuff from a mile away. (as cited in Melberg Schwier, 1990, pp. 28–29)

Sometimes, the requirements of a system to provide services for people living in institutions en masse meant that drastic measures were taken with long-lasting results. Some of these systemic conveniences led to procedures on and practices with residents—such as the use of completely puréed food diets—that would affect their enjoyment of mealtimes for the rest of their lives. Although such diets have sometimes been used to reduce the risk of choking, they are not typically justifiable because these diets cause other health problems and increase the risk of aspiration, which may also be life threatening (Lowman, 2004). Stewart Howard described what happened to his older brother, Oliver, who lives in a residential facility in South Australia:

> *It must have been 30 years ago when all of Ollie's teeth were extracted in the institution. They told Mum about it later. It never really twigged with me until I talked to other family members of people where he lives and there were such a large number of residents who had false teeth or needed them. I realized that a number of people must have had all their teeth taken out back then. I suppose that is what happened so they didn't have to be concerned about dental problems. But since Ollie had no teeth, it was assumed for years that he could only eat puréed food. But we found when we took him out with us that he loved hamburgers as long as we cut them up small. I eventually got someone to follow up, so now he has more solid foods at the institution. It's just that nobody had ever explored it.*

Not all people with disabilities will need physical assistance with eating.

Learning from the Past

The intent of looking back is not to simply vilify past practices, but it's difficult to fully understand the importance of nurturing quality connections and mealtimes without understanding the past. For one, history can repeat itself. As Ebenezer Scrooge found out, only by understanding the past can one embrace a better future.

A Spot of Tea Goes a Long Way

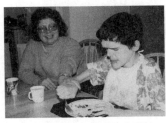

A light hand on Angela's wrist is a gentle reminder to slow down.

Angie had developed a lot of institutional behavior [after 25 years], you know, like grabbing food at meals so nobody would take it from her. Here, at mealtime, the staff sit down with [the residents] and chat about the day and what they might do tomorrow. If Angie starts eating too fast, a staff [member] will gently put her hand on Angie's and reassure her that she doesn't have to eat so fast. Isn't that wonderful? I spoke to a staff person named Susan and she said not to worry [about Angie's long history of wandering at night]. She and Angela were up, having a cup of Chamomile tea to relax. I thought that was wonderful. Isn't that a much nicer way to look at our children? She's not a *behavior problem* because she won't sleep; she just needs a nice cup of tea! Maybe what was seen as a behavior problem was really [her] trying to tell us something. (as cited in Melberg Schwier, 1996, p. 7)

THE QUALITY OF "THE INGREDIENTS"

The ingredients that come to mind when we think about quality mealtimes for people with and without disabilities go far beyond the food itself. The food, really, is a good excuse to be with one another for a time. Those strictly task-oriented souls who measure the success of time spent together in terms of the nutritionally balanced meal or the perfect soufflé may miss out on the true richness and texture of human relationship. To go beyond the basics of a mealtime experience can mean a deeper appreciation for the "quality ingredients" that exist in the people present, not just the food. This is a notion that good cooks, good diners, and good restaurateurs all understand.

James Schwier, our brother-in-law/uncle, established Whisky's, an upscale restaurant in Lawrenceburg, Indiana, in 1985. Today, it serves as a place where people go when they want a nice evening out and a quality dining experience. Schwier encourages his wait staff to become not only knowledgeable but also prideful of the dishes they are serving to their customers. Schwier says:

Selling the food creates so much of the ambiance for our guests. Our servers must know their product, appreciate its quality, and be able to honestly recommend it to diners. For our regular customers, the wait staff know what they like and remember that so they can help make the dining experience something special. To know the customer, to appreciate and remember their preferences, and to make them feel special, is everything.

Knowing the people involved—to "know the customer"—and to look beyond stereotypes and reputations, means everything in terms of fostering a relationship between people with and without disabilities, too:

> We were made to feel. The concept of *touch,* started at birth, grows from something physical to something emotional. Have you ever been out for a dinner with a friend and had him or her sit across from the table from you? Over the course of dinner you become wrapped up in a conversation, so much so that the rest of the world disappears and the only people who are there in the restaurant are the two of you. You feel embraced, but you never touch physically. We need to look at how people learn to show intimacy in ways that are quite abstract. (Melberg Schwier & Hingsburger, 2000, p. 27)

Table Manners

Being in tune with another person is easier if we do a good job of looking at the world from her perspective. Putting yourself into the shoes of someone with a disability sounds like a pretty simple, common-sense approach to many people. People can make a conscious effort to try to experience the world in different ways, like those participating in the activities or simulations described later in this chapter, but it doesn't always work. One of the reasons it doesn't may stem from the fact that there are some people who simply do not accept that a person with a disability is *like them.*

In Bogdan and Taylor's *Inside Out: The Social Meaning of Mental Retardation,* the authors suggested that people create a way of viewing individuals with disabilities as human beings either like themselves or other than themselves. In the former, every thought and action stems from the foundational belief that all people are considered under the umbrella term of *we*—and therefore deserving of equality, dignity, and the elements of life we all enjoy. Or, according to the latter, people who have differences are considered as *them,* beings who can never be related to in a way that allows them to be part of the same human family. To make people with disabilities separate from the rest of humanity provides some people a sense of relief, perhaps, that they are "not one of us" (Bogdan & Taylor, 1982, p. 14).

Gill Rutherford is the coordinator of disability studies at the Dunedin College of Education/Te Kura Akau Taitoka, in New Zealand. She encourages students to look within to clarify their own beliefs about themselves and their fellow human beings. To merely become competent in the basic, practical skills of care is just a matter of learning the mechanics of human services. That shouldn't be good enough. She notes:

Without a sound understanding, and an appreciation for the gifts of another human being, you're just tinkering with someone's life. I think you can actually do things that are harmful. If you see this person as someone very different from you and as just a job, then mealtime just means your job is getting food into him. You just feed him. I've seen animals being fed with more grace than some people.

Rutherford says there are many wonderful examples of staff in residential services who believe mealtime is an opportunity to develop relationships. Eating is a basic, everyday activity that can provide many opportunities for undivided attention and support. But she fears that people who believe these times are for sharing food and each other are still exceptions to the rule. We've all experienced the uncomfortable, frustrating moments when we wait for a store clerk or server to make eye contact and acknowledge our presence even as we hand over the money or wave a hand to order. It's as though we don't exist. We, however, have the option of complaining or leaving. Many people living within service systems do not have this option. The dignity for people who live in services is in how they are supported in the ordinary things of life. If you are someone with a disability, having your food shoveled into you by a staff person who doesn't even sit down because she is talking to another staff person about what she did on the weekend, complaining about her wages, or worse, talking about other people with disabilities, you enjoy no dignity or respect.

Rutherford teaches students who will go on to be teacher aids and support staff in human services. Although serving people at mealtime isn't taught formally, she often uses it as a way to look at support strategies and attitudes. Rutherford tells her students:

If the situation is such that one person has all of the control and is feeding someone who is powerless, the first person is getting the job of providing nutrition done, but they are missing out on so much more. If you are someone who needs help to get food to your mouth, having some choice about who does that and how is so important, yet rarely acknowledged. Mealtime can be as intimate as bathing if a person needs a lot of support. Think of how it would feel to depend on another person you don't know, or may not even like, for such a personal act. Think how a mealtime must feel if you suspect that person may not really care about you as a human being.

Many people find the question of bib use to be a quandary. On the one hand, some people who have difficulty managing food and eating have found bibs helpful in protecting their clothing. On the other hand, the worry is that bibs detract from someone's dignity. Clothing protectors or aprons look less infantile. For anyone who's not an infant, avoid cartoon characters and juvenile designs. When helping someone eat, don't use the bib to wipe the person's mouth. That's what a napkin is for. And never leave a soiled bib, clothing protector, or apron on someone after a meal.

 If adapted utensils are needed, respect the person's age and dignity. Look for the most age-appropriate options. A Winnie-the-Pooh tippy cup is fine for a 3-year-old, but what does it say about a 30-year-old?

An Italian Who Doesn't Enjoy Food? *Impossibile!*

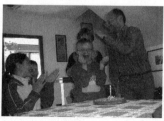

Nothing says excitement like candles on your own birthday cake. Andrea shows his appreciation with brother Luca, dad Enrico, and friends Claudia and Fabio.

Andrea has Down syndrome. Nonna, his grandmother, worries and fusses over him. She worries that he doesn't eat very much; it is only within the last couple of months that Andrea will tolerate anything more than yogurt and gelato. I say, as long as he is healthy and is eating some good food, why push? He will eat when he is ready. Coming to the table for a meal is not only about eating. —Edi Cecchini, Italy

It is hard for me to realize that it is possible to be a member of our family and to imagine one does not like food. That there is no real interest in it. This is impossible if you are Italian. But Andrea simply did not have the interest, so we did not want to turn it into a problem. —Enrico Barone, Italy

 If people aren't hungry, they shouldn't be forced to eat. People shouldn't feel forced to clean their plates. Offer the possibility of putting food away to warm up later.

In our society, it's acceptable to cut food at the table for small children. If you or your meal partner still requires the food to be cut up but would be embarrassed by this assistance, why not do the cutting in the kitchen before presenting it at the table? If you're dining out, make the request of the server when you order. An adult with dignity intact can manage a sliced chicken breast or a de-boned and sliced pork chop.

Undivided attention can be one of the most precious gifts we can give to and receive from another person. It is possibly one of the strongest forms of acknowledgement that says, "You are important to me." Pat Katz, Canadian author and time management consultant, insists that despite our protests, time is something we all have, it's just that some fail to recognize the power of even a small gift of it to another person. That gift can be given—and received—during mealtime. She adds:

Sitting face to face, knee to knee, eye to eye, and ignoring all else says, 'I'm here. I'm yours.' It's a kind of focus and surrender that builds relationships in a way that all the multitasking in the world never will.

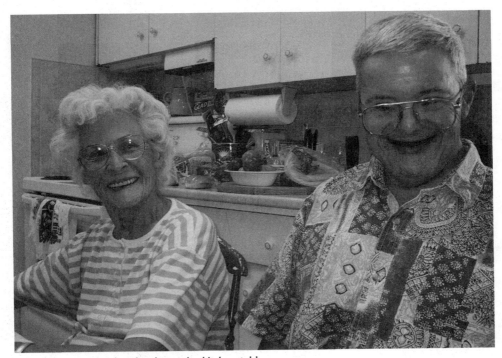

Marg and son Dale plan the day at the kitchen table.

Alfred Uhry adapted his 1987 play *Driving Miss Daisy* for the motion picture of the same name (Fini Zanuck & Beresford, 1989), a story of human connection and respect based on his own southern Jewish grandmother and her African American driver. Gill Rutherford, who teaches disabilities studies, makes the final few seconds of the movie required viewing for her students. In the final scene, Hoke (played by Morgan Freeman), now much older, has come to visit Miss Daisy (Jessica Tandy), who is living in the nursing home and in ill health. "Now look here. You haven't eaten your Thanksgiving pie," he observes. With trembling hands, she tries to pick up her fork. Tenderly, he offers, "Here. Let me help you. . ." As he gently helps her to taste her pumpkin pie, the love, gratitude, and respect each has for the other creates a sweet connection that is arguably one of the most respectful and delicate human interactions captured on film. Without exception, Rutherford says, as her students come to understand the profound difference between feeding and dining, some are moved to tears.

HOW DOES IT FEEL?

According to Dianne Koontz Lowman (2004), in the best instances, meals provide children with the nutrition needed for growth and survival, pleasures from the senses, opportunities for positive social interaction, and ways to increase independence in eating and eating skills. This isn't always the case, unfortunately. According to Orelove and Sobsey, "Some children and adults struggle through seemingly endless meals with little opportunity for positive social interaction or learning, desperately trying to obtain adequate foods and fluids without choking or gagging" (1996, p. 301).

 Some people with cerebral palsy who have more muscle involvement can expend a lot of energy in the daily struggle to control muscle coordination. Learn the person's preferences as to how much support he wants to receive. Something you think is an important task, like eating unassisted, may be too exhausting for the person to manage for a whole meal.

 If you are helping someone to eat, pay close attention to the person's breathing patterns. A forkful of food shouldn't be presented during an inhale or exhale, but rather, just before either.

 Make sure you are at the same level as the person or slightly lower when helping him eat so he isn't looking upward and hyper-extending his neck.

Living the Golden Rule

If you are just getting to know someone with a disability, whether that person is a family member or a potential friend, pay attention to his interactions with others. Ask questions. Listen and observe and use the old but always useful Golden Rule, "Do unto others as you would have them do unto you," as your guide. Think about what is happening. Beyond that, feel what is happening. Think carefully about your own mealtime experiences. Take a good look and ask yourself, "If this were me, is this how I would want to be treated?"

 If someone cannot physically manage to wipe his or her own mouth during the meal, ask if you can assist. Don't swoop in, push the person's head back, and wipe. Without fuss and with dignity, ask if you may help, and then say what you're going to do. Then wipe with a napkin—firmly but gently—and start at the side of the person's mouth.

Institutional rules don't always have a great grasp on reality. Don't be afraid to ask "why" when confronted with a rule that doesn't seem to make sense or flies in the face of promoting dignity or good health. Just because something "has always been done" doesn't mean it needs to be done. Watch out for "us" and "them" statements. These types of comments may be red flags that may indicate that the speaker views people with disabilities as different, perhaps even less than human, and, therefore, less deserving of respect and equal treatment. Here are some other red flag statements:

- "It really doesn't matter. She'll eat anything."
- "You have to really be firm and insist that he eat it, otherwise he just sits there."
- "If he makes too much noise, take the plate away."
- "She gets really cranky halfway through a meal, but just ignore it. She just wants attention."
- "She's not allowed in the kitchen; she tried helping once and cut herself, so the kitchen is out of bounds."
- "Just take him to McDonald's. He wouldn't really appreciate a nice restaurant anyway."

Nicola Schaefer, whose daughter Catherine has significant "inconveniences," as Nicola calls them, including quadriplegia and lack of speech, has always been mindful of surrounding her daughter with people who appreciate her. That includes not only seeing her as a "beautiful, thoughtful young woman" but also having a sense of partnership as Catherine is supported to live a full, interesting life. Catherine does not speak and relies on other people for all of her needs, including intimate care. She lives in a cooperative housing arrangement. Schaefer recalls one young woman who was thinking of moving into the house with Catherine:

> She asked all sorts of questions about how Catherine ate, what sorts of foods she liked. We talked about her tendency to get blocked up from time to time. An enema is sometimes the only way out, so to speak. This young woman left and, on the way home, bought one of those enema kits you can buy at the drugstore. At her apartment, she asked her girlfriend if she'd be willing to give her an enema so she could really see how it felt. She told me later that if she was going to be giving one, even once, to Catherine, the least she could do would be to have a good idea of what it felt like. I thought, "Right, you're hired. You're brilliant."

Understanding how it feels to receive intimate care is important. Shirley Gerein is a residential director of a group home agency. Support staff in group homes for seniors with disabilities such as the ones she manages need to find out what life really feels like to be a resident so that they can understand how their attitude and care affects the recipient. Staff can make sure people are not only comfortable but also that their remaining years are dignified. Gerein requires her staff to be blindfolded while they experience a ground-up diet. They are paired up, and one assists the other to eat. Experiencing the texture of puréed hamburger or how it feels to have someone scrape food off your lips and chin with a spoon helps support people make many small decisions each day about how they treat other people.

 Have a manageable number of food items during a meal. Some people can be overwhelmed with too many choices and decisions.

Ultimately, whether the consumption of food and drink is a feeding or dining experience depends largely on what people bring to the table emotionally and philosophically. Those who have experienced mealtime in less than ideal conditions are perhaps the most appreciative of the act of sharing good food with willing people in convivial surroundings.

Pay attention to the table setting. For some people who have perception and visual difficulties, a white plate, a clear glass, silver cutlery, and a white napkin on a white tablecloth may "disappear." Try arranging light-colored foods such as potatoes and pasta on a dark-colored plate, for example, so there is a contrast.

 Use clear or translucent cups with a person who needs assistance to drink so you can see when the fluid reaches his mouth. Iced tea up the nose isn't pleasant.

ACTIVITIES

The following are three simple yet powerful sensitizing exercises to help caregivers experience the emotions, physical reactions, and implications of the fundamental differences between feeding and dining. They will allow you to stop for a moment and put yourself in someone else's shoes—or in this case, put yourself at someone else's plate.

Simulations like these help us understand how "exquisitely intimate the relationship is" when we share a mealtime with someone (J. Zgola, personal communication, 2003). And if you still need more convincing about the difference between feeding and dining, answer this: What do we call the room in our homes where we share meals together? It's the dining room, not the feeding room.

Feed Me or Dine Me

This exercise, courtesy of author and consultant Dave Hingsburger, is helpful in comparing the different moods created when a mealtime is viewed as a job or as an enriching opportunity to be with another person. Is it a communal, human act of nurturing and togetherness or a rote act of feeding time at the zoo? How does each participant—the person feeding and the person being fed feel? Embarrassed? Uncomfortable? Intimidated? Intimidating? Nurtured? Cared for? Cared about? Inhuman? Inhumane? Inconsequential? Loved? This exercise should give participants a close-up and hands-on feel for what it might be like.

1. Choose a food item; dry cookies work well and don't create an unnecessary mess. Check for food allergies among participants. Have participants wash their hands.

2. Ask participants to pair up. Identify one as person A, who has a disability wherein he or she can't speak, can't use his or her hands, and requires total care and as-

sistance including assistance to eat. Identify the other person as B, the one who will provide the assistance. B comes up to get a cookie.

3. B is instructed to "feed A the cookie." Allow this to go on for a few minutes to make sure A gets a couple of bites.

4. Stop the activity and ask A what the experience was like. Then ask A, "What would be the qualities of a good feeder?" Use those terms. What generally happens is that people start to change the terms from "being fed" and "feeder" as they talk about wanting to feel included, needing to know that B isn't disgusted by what they're doing, that they're being talked to and looked at. They want it to be a so- cial human interaction, so it becomes very clear that this isn't just making sure a person gets some food, but rather, that it is an intimate interaction with another person.

5. Now have A come up for a cookie and switch roles so that B is the one eating. After a few minutes, stop the activity and have B describe the experience.

What we always see is a substantive change in the mood in the room. There's now a gentle murmur as people are talking. The As are describing what they're doing; they're describing what B is eating. They're physically close. It really changes the whole experience. What people come to really understand and appreciate is that when we have these opportunities to be with someone sharing food, we have the chance to do something together that isn't medical or clinical. It isn't just getting nutrition into a body that's different from yours. It's not a job. It's more about creating a social envi- ronment. For so many people with disabilities, that food may be the most pleasurable experience they have in their day. "And just think—you've waited all day for this food," Hingsburger says. "You've looked forward to it, and here's someone just shoving it in without acknowledging that it's even enjoyable for you. What's that about?"

 Allergies and asthma can produce a variety of unpleasant sensations. Coughing, sneezing, and gasping can cause serious problems such as aspiration (inhaling small amounts of food and liquid into the lungs) at mealtime. Be aware of how to minimize these difficulties; talk to the person, her family, and her caregivers to learn strategies that work.

Time Trials

This exercise reminds us of how power is so easily removed from someone with a disability. The intent should be to experience the feelings that come when others don't give enough time and support to someone eating a meal and what it feels like when others take away a person's opportunity to contribute to the preparation of a meal. The exercise reminds participants that mealtime, whether preparing or eating a meal, is a social experience, not a job to hurry through.

The task will be to make a peanut butter and jelly sandwich in 30 seconds.

1.   Gather materials. You will need a knife, a stopwatch or timer, sliced bread, jelly or jam, and peanut butter. (Ensure no one has peanut butter allergies. If so, just use the jelly or jam.) Have participants wash their hands.

2.   Ask participants to pair up. Identify one as A (a person with a disability) and the other as B (a staff person or caregiver).

3.   Tell A that he or she is the sandwich maker. Tell B that he or she is of the vocal opinion that A is not fast enough, is not doing the task the right way, and is making a mess. Explain the task, set the timer, and begin.

4.   After 30 seconds, stop the exercise and have A and B switch roles.

5.   Ask A and B to describe their feelings in each role.

6.   Ask A and B to switch roles and begin again. This time, there is no time limit. A and B are two people who happen to want to make sandwiches. They may work together on one sandwich or they may each make one. They will announce when they have completed the task. Ask A and B to describe their feelings in the second experience.

You can create variations of this (you might have one person in the pair take control and cut the food for the other, wipe his or her face, control what food is eaten next, and decide when the meal is finished).

What can you do if you're cooking, baking, or eating a meal and the bowl or dish won't stay still? Cut out a piece of Dycem, a nonsticky sheeting that grips on both sides. Dycem comes in small pieces, as place mats, or in rolls so you can cut to the desired length and shape. You can try plastic cupboard lining, too; it's in the kitchen supply aisle of the supermarket. Put it underneath while you're stirring or eating to keep the bowl or plate from sliding away. A word of caution: Dycem and other nonskid materials can be made of latex, and some people have an allergy to this. Plastic liners are a good way to avoid reactions, but in general, do pay attention to skin allergies as well as to food allergies.

Two Powerful Fingers

This exercise is from Jitka Zgola. A simple simulation shows the importance of helping someone retain even a small measure of control.

1. Ask participants to pair up. Identify one as A and the other as B. Each has a lollipop. (In Zgola & Bordillon, 2001, a glass of water is used for this exercise.)

2. Instruct B to sit on his or her hands. B has no verbal communication. A is to unwrap the lollipop and feed it to B. A should let B lick the lollipop three or four times.

3. Stop the exercise. Ask B how this feels. People generally say here that the problem is a lack of any control. They're really at the mercy of A. When the lollipop is thrust into their mouth, they can't easily get rid of it short of trying to spit it out. But with A holding it in place, that's difficult. Then when B does want more, A pulls it away.

4. After some discussion, ask the pairs to try a different way of handling the experience. B still cannot hold the lollipop, but this time, B sits on only one hand. This time, B can use two fingers of her free hand to rest them on A's hand that is holding the lollipop. Try the exercise again.

5. After a few minutes, ask how it feels. This time, even with the slightest pressure, B can indicate with just two fingers that he wants the lollipop out, whether he wants more, or where he wants it in his mouth. The mealtime becomes a more balanced sharing rather than only one person being in charge.

6. Switch roles and repeat the exercise so that both people get a chance to experience it.

7. Ask participants how the experience changed when they were able to exert just a little control.

Zgola poses an interesting thought: A little bit is infinitely more than nothing. "If we take everything away from a person, they have nothing," she says. "But if we help them hold on to even the tiniest 'anything' they can possibly manage, we give them access to infinitely more." If you are assisting someone who requires a lot of support to eat and you are helping the person retain even a little bit of control, it makes a huge difference.

 When you are assisting someone who requires a lot of support to eat his or meal, you are, in essence, replacing the person's hand to eat (Zgola, personal communication, 2003). Sitting kitty-corner is useful for comfortable contact and hand movement.

One's mouth and hands work better when one's trunk and shoulders have a firm base of support. A footrest helps. So does a lap tray or a table; it's not just a place to put the plate but a helpful foundation for elbows to stabilize the neck and head.

 Use your own body to give support to someone if needed to help the person get into a comfortable position for eating. Each person is unique, so a pillow or wedge that works well for one person may not work for someone else.

 Pay attention to how a person is sitting for a meal. Sitting straight and comfortably with feet on the floor makes it easier for someone to use his or her arms and to swallow properly.

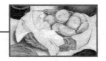

CHAPTER 3

Mealtime in Purgatory

BARB HANDAHL

I started working for the State of Minnesota at the Faribault State School and Hospital in March of 1968. I was 18 years old. After graduation from high school in 1967, I went to Business College. I didn't care for it, so, being born and raised in Faribault, I came back home and started working at the institution for people with intellectual disabilities, following in my grandmother's footsteps. She worked at the institution in the sewing room for 10 years.

The School for Idiots and Imbeciles opened in 1879 and closed in 1998 as the Faribault Regional Center. The moment I stepped foot on the grounds of the Faribault State School and Hospital, as it was called in 1968, I knew I had entered another world, a strange and unfamiliar world to me as a young girl. I was sent to "Psychiatric Technician" class for 6 months. We had to wear all white uniforms. We were told that if our shoelaces were not immaculately white, it was the same as wearing dirty underwear. First names were not allowed, ever. I was called Dube, my last name then, and if I wanted to speak with Marge Johnson, I was to say "Johnson," not even "Miss" or "Mrs." I was trained to take care of people's physical needs.

One of the first buildings that I worked in as a psychiatric technician was home to many people with low cognitive abilities who were nonambulatory. Some of the people who lived there were called the "bed patients," and at that time in the late 1960s, very rarely were these people gotten out of bed. Not even for meals. I do remember as time went by there came about a policy stating that everyone had to be in a sitting position out of bed when they were being fed. After that, people were gotten out of bed to eat their meals, only to sit next to their bed in their wheelchairs to be fed their food.

All of these people needed to be fed because they did not have the ability to feed themselves, and there were not sufficient staff or time to teach them these skills or let

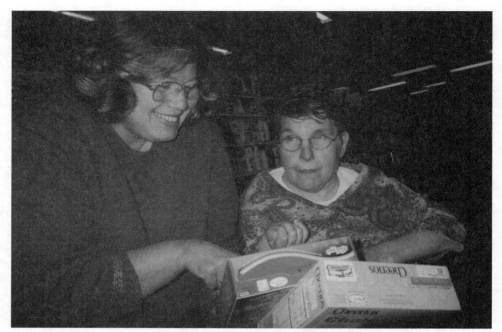

Barb (left) and CeCe do some comparison shopping at the local grocery.

them participate at some level. The food was all puréed, and it was a matter of strictly feeding and changing people one after another as quickly as possible. There were about 15 people and two staff usually taking care of the "bed patients." As I reflect, it could not have been pleasant for people as it was always hurry up and get done. Get everyone fed and cleaned up; that was the goal. No personal time, no quiet music, no laughing, smiling, telling stories, not even any talk about the Minnesota weather, just get the job done.

In another part of this building there were 36 "patients" who lived on two connecting units. A few, maybe six people, were labeled the "self-feeders." They were taken to the dining room ahead of time and set up at tables with their food. Then the assembly line started with the remaining people, and that's what it was, an assembly line. Outside the dining room everyone was lined up sitting in his or her wheelchair in a long hall. They waited for their turn to be wheeled into the dining room to be fed. All staff available were used to feed the people. I even think sometimes the janitors or the laundry ladies would come and help us feed if we were running behind schedule. After each meal the dining room was mopped and the kitchen area was hosed down. Of course, cleaning had to be done according to a time schedule; that was the reason the janitors would come and help us feed.

I can remember standing directly in front of the person holding a bowl of mush and basically feeding one spoonful after another as quickly as the person would swallow. There's even a photo of me doing just that on a hospital brochure showing our "state of the art care" at that time. The main objective was to get this person fed so the next person could eat. I can remember even feeding two people at one time on days when we were short staffed. The dining room was very noisy and the conversation amongst staff—over the heads of the people we were feeding—usually consisted about what we were going to do for our lunch or where we were going shopping to catch the latest sale after work. This was the only time when all staff were together since we were spread out in the building during the day doing our own work in various settings.

I guess people really didn't see that mealtimes could be a special time in a person's life. We didn't think about engaging those we cared for in any of the process, other than thinking that feeding was a task to be completed three times a day. I think that is just the tell-tale story of institutional life at that time.

As the years went by and as philosophies about people with disabilities changed, little by little by little, life began to get better. When the functional movement took place in the late 1970s, large dining rooms disappeared. Smaller settings for mealtimes were designed. Day programs and assistive technology came into existence and people were beginning to be supported to learn how to feed themselves and to use special dinnerware to assist them to be more independent.

People did not go to large dining rooms, but remained in their day program or classrooms to eat their lunch or had their meals in smaller settings back on their units. I remember that hot dogs and peanut butter were prohibited because there were incidents where people choked on these foods and one person died.

However, the food now came on individual insulated trays from one main kitchen. Oh boy, what a great plastic smell that was to be enjoyed when the tray cover was lifted off. Staff were to now role model social skills, so trays of food were sent so the staff could eat with the people, too. Most of the time staff did not want to eat, as the food was not very appetizing. Sometimes the cold food was hot and the hot food cold. Of course, when the food came pre-measured in individual servings on these plastic insulated trays, there was never an opportunity for a person to have a second helping, if by chance someone would want one.

When the normalization principle hit the campus in the early 1980s, the living units in the institution were changed into more apartment-like settings with still fewer people living in them. And again, we changed the mealtime settings. People no longer ate in their classrooms but had to leave their classroom or dayroom and go to a "normal" dining room. Still, the food came served in individualized plastic trays. I can recall that special meals were planned where people did get to cook now and then or be a part of meal preparation. That was a real treat. It was a treat to do what most people take for granted as part of everyday normal life.

In 1991 I left the institution and started working in a state-operated group home where six people lived. I work there today. We still have many rules we have to follow, but we are continually working hard to actually support people to live a life in which each person has control of his own life. After living in the community now for 12 years, one of the men in the home where I work says his favorite food still is hot dogs and now he actually gets to eat them. Everyone enjoys peanut butter, too.

The people I support love going grocery shopping. Often they may see an old staff person from the institution or a new friend they have made since living in the community. They like to stop and chat. The grocery store is a great social setting. The people I work with love planning their meals and having a part in the preparation, too. They also get to invite the neighbors over to enjoy afternoon coffee and treats. And they enjoy going to neighbors' homes, too, for the same.

For people who have high health needs such as those I worked with when I first started at the institution, they too now live in homes of four to six people. They get to go grocery shopping and have an active part in the food preparation. The food for some of these individuals may still be in a puréed state, but it is home-cooked and people get to take part in their own meal preparations in whatever way they can. And if they are not able to actively help, they can supervise and watch the activity while enjoying the great smells of food being cooked in their own kitchen at home.

As I think back over 30 years, I see that I went through the same changes as the people who had been institutionalized. As a young girl, I only knew what I was taught at that time. Once I was freed from the institution and was able to work in the community, I realized how we treated people. How restricted, devalued, and isolated their lives were. I went from being a staff member who provided service *to* a person to a staff member who now provides support *for* a person. Today, I support people to have control over their own lives. And if they want to go to a restaurant for supper, change the menu, bake their favorite chocolate chip cookies, have pancakes for supper, or have a friend over for a meal, I make that happen. We are all so much happier in life and better off because of it. Had we only given as much attention to the dignity of people during mealtime as we did to the condition of our shoelaces, people would have had better lives.

A BALANCED DIET

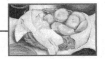

CHAPTER 4

Mealtime as a
Chance to Refocus

*The joys of the table belong equally to all ages,
conditions, countries and times; they mix with all other
pleasures, and remain the last to console us for their loss.*
—Jean-Anthelme Brillat-Savarin

An unwritten (or too often written) assumption is that any activity in the life of someone with a disability has to have some sort of therapeutic benefit. Families and caregivers must be vigilant to ensure that ordinary, everyday activities like mealtimes
remain just that—ordinary and everyday.

LEARNING TO APPRECIATE THE ORDINARY

In *Circles of Friends: People with Disabilities and Their Friends Enrich the Lives of One
Another,* Robert Perske wrote,

> Mark Twain once said that any time you can get your hands on a modifier, you
> should kill it. Maybe the time has come to go after the adjective *special* every time
> it is used to describe people with disabilities [and the services set up for them]:
> special education, special educators, special classrooms, special recreation, special
> buses, special . . . classes . . . when you hear special used this way, grab it by the
> throat and do it in. (1988, p. 59)

We don't want to make mealtimes *special* in the way Perske laments. We like to
think of the mealtime experience in terms of *fusion cuisine*. There is no one correct

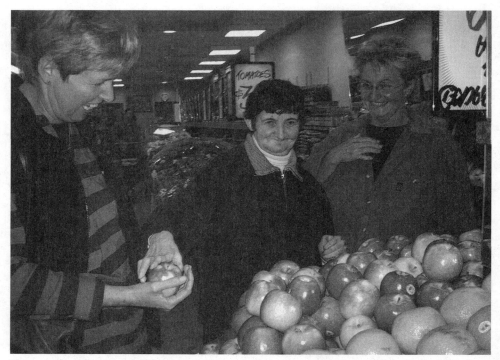

Sisters Beth and Margie and friend Jan admire the produce as part of their afternoon trip to the shops in North Sydney.

recipe for enjoying mealtime with someone else; there is no one correct meal and there is no one correct circumstance. Some common elements should come into play, however, such as getting to know the individual with a disability—his likes, dislikes, health concerns, if any, adaptations that might make mealtimes easier, and cultural traditions or religious beliefs. We hope that family members, friends, next-door neighbors, and the people who work in human services to support people with disabilities in their daily lives will use any or all of these elements of mealtime as a way to connect—to fuse—with someone who has a disability. With so few opportunities for intimate friendships outside of the service system, people with disabilities "have little chance of disproving the stereotypes" (Bogdan & Biklen, 1977, p. 14). We don't think this has changed to the extent we'd like. We believe mealtimes can be a great social equalizer and one of the best ways to see an individual as he is, not as a "patient," "client," or "one of them."

When someone with a disability has a job that puts her before the public as a capable and friendly person, it helps others appreciate the person beyond the stereotype. Raffath Sayeed, whose son has a disability, notes how his son's active, contributing presence in the community has helped stereotypes to crumble:

> *He's a most gregarious guy. He's working at a restaurant now and he knows everybody. He's a busboy, a greeter, and they tell me he welcomes people*

and he goes to check to see if they're enjoying their meal. That's not really part of his job, but he sees what should be done and he'll do it. Sometimes he'll watch and he'll go back to see if people want dessert. People ask him what he'd recommend, so he makes suggestions. Someone said the name of the restaurant should be Rashaad's, not Ricky's.

RESPECT EVERYDAY FAMILY LIFE

Many parents of children with disabilities bemoan the fact that their lives are often dictated by therapies and programs. They have concerns like these:

- *Why can't professionals understand we need to be a family? My child just needs to be a child now and then.*
- *Why does everything have to focus on the disability?*
- *If I did everything the OT {occupational therapist} and physio {physical therapist} told me, I would spend 3 to 4 hours at every meal, feeding my child.*

Families must be able to make some distinctions between professional interventions that may be necessary to support their child's growth and development and living life as an ordinary family. It's disconcerting enough that people with disabilities can't go for a swim without it being "aqua therapy" or ride a horse without it being "equine therapy." People with disabilities don't go to the grocery or the farmer's market; they have "life skills training" or "community access." Of course, we're being facetious—but not much. Not that these disability-directed activities are a bad thing, but for someone with a disability, it might be nice to make a meal, go out for lunch, or go to a neighbor's for coffee without showing up as a tick mark on a clipboard.

Sometimes a therapeutic name is tied to funding, and families do understand more than ever that a person's disability is the reason why a professional is needed in the first place. Still, a disability really is a small part of who that person is—a significant part, certainly, but only a part. What is needed is a profound shift in perspective. Is the question, "What kind of program can we put someone in?" or should it be, "What kind of life can we build for this person?"

Occupational therapist Jitka Zgola consults with residential facilities on making mealtime more enjoyable. She suggests that instead of seeing mealtime as just another activity to complete in order to move onto more important things, we can look at the benefits of mealtime as a rich opportunity to experience the senses. In a very ordinary way, it can serve the purposes of therapy without appearing as a medical model:

It has always given me pause to think that we rush through mealtime in 10 minutes so we can get cleaned up and move on to the next thing on the agenda. Then the activities staff person has to come up with all sorts of exercises to offer sensory stimulation. Why can't the activities person have lunch with people for a half hour in a nice, quiet, intensely intimate spot and enjoy exquisitely stimulating food like liver paté on crackers and raspberry cordial on shaved ice? Doesn't that make more sense? Can't we be creative?

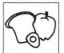 Have you ever been seated in a restaurant only to have the server ignore you? When he finally does arrive, water glasses are slammed down and specials mumbled in a way you don't understand. Did you get the feeling the server would rather you just got up and left and quit bothering him? Contrast that with your best dining experience. Mealtimes can feel like a frantic assembly line for people with disabilities. Remember to make the experience a memorable one.

Sometimes, an ordinary outing for a meal should be just that. Robert Perske recalled his days as a chaplain at an institution for people with disabilities in Topeka, Kansas:

One time, I thought I'd take five or maybe six guys—the men who were helping me keep the chapel clean—out for sort of a thank you dinner. We pile into my car and off we go for a steak dinner, my treat. Once we ordered, I found out that not one of them knew how to cut a steak. They'd never had one. Grown men, never had a steak before. And it really kind of bothered me because I didn't want this to be some sort of teaching, life skills lesson. I was just hoping us men would go out and have a good time. Made me kinda sad.

The everyday occupation of meal preparation and sharing is an adult activity that garners respect. It also paves the way for social interactions with others. What are the implications of this occupation of daily life and how does being involved in this "work" affect self-esteem and confidence?

Helping Is a Part of Life

Dorothy wouldn't be able to go and make a cake herself, mainly because she can't read well enough. She couldn't manage the recipe. But if you have staff who do all the cooking and clearing up for people who have disabilities, doing all the thinking, then that's not really normal, day-to-day living, is it? I suppose adults with a disability who didn't know how to make themselves a sandwich would be missing out on that enjoyment. I suppose Mum and Dad would have thought about the bigger picture for Dorothy. It would have been easier for Mum just to do it herself. But Dorothy was always expected to get up and make herself a sandwich if she needed to, just like the rest of us. —Robyn Hadfield, Australia

The Cake

A guy came back to the community after living in an institution for many years. I was working on the staff in a group home then. I remember being there at Phil's annual IPP [individual program plan] where he was asked what his goals were. It was really sad because he said his goal was that he wanted his mother to love him. He felt that she'd just left him in the institution and hadn't visited him. True, she was visiting him a bit now because he lived close by, but she was very uncomfortable with him and the visits were always very short. Anyway, so here we are in this group home and we knew her birthday was coming up and we asked Phil if he wanted to buy her a card.

"No," he said, which really surprised us because he'd do anything for his mom. But then he said no, he didn't want to buy her a card. "I want to bake her a cake." He'd never cooked or baked before, but this was something he really wanted to do because people got cakes on their birthdays.

So we make this happen. I'm sitting at the kitchen table. It seems like everything he ever touches or looks at just falls apart. So my friend Bob offers to help make this cake with him. Why Bob doesn't pick a simple recipe, I have no idea, but the one they pick calls for scalded milk. So he's got the pot and they measure out the milk and dump it into the pot. The pot is on the counter to be transferred to the stovetop.

Bob says, "Okay, we have to get all our ingredients out so we have everything we need. So we need to get the flour." Okay, well, the flour is kept up in the cupboard over the counter. So Phil gets up on a chair to reach for the flour. Just as he reaches for the bag, the pot handle gets caught in his belt loop on the way up. Phil feels it, swings around taking the pot with him. The milk cascades in an arc across the room. He's startled, loses his grip on the bag of flour, which falls on his head and splits open, sending a cloudburst of flour over him and all over the rest of the kitchen. As the flour settles in the silence, he stands there on the chair, blinking, his face completely white. He stands looking at us and we stand looking at him. He asks fearfully, and I quote, "Do I *have* to get the eggs?" Well, it was hysterical, and we burst out laughing. The thing was, the moment we started to laugh, he knew he wasn't in trouble. The more we laughed, the more he laughed until you could see the little rivers of tears running through the flour down his cheeks. We cleaned everything up and laughed for about another hour. He ended up making a fine cake, a different one, but we had the best time. Things don't have to be perfect! It seems that people with disabilities are never allowed to make mistakes because that somehow reflects on us and on our teaching abilities. "My God, what will people think of my parenting/teaching/support skills if this person messes up?" But we have to just lighten up. Life is supposed to be fun. —David Hingsburger, Canada.

Do you know someone who has trouble reaching and grabbing? Reachers with grasping ends operated by a simple trigger mechanism help people reach for things on the ground and on lower shelves. Emphasize to someone with a disability that, when shopping, it is still important to ask store employees, family members, and friends for help in reaching heavier items up high.

Do you know someone who likes to bake? If you find those crank sifters too hard to manage, battery-operated flour sifters eliminate the need to turn the crank.

Try using electric can openers that sit on the counter. If cans are hard to open, all this requires is that you hold the can up to the magnet and push a button.

The Food Escape

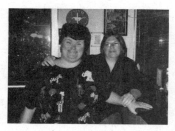

Laura and Rory at a favorite haunt.

Both of us like to eat, and it seems like it's a relaxing time. We don't see each other every day or every week, so when we do get together two or three times a month, we like to go out. It's a lot more meaningful to be together out in the world, in the regular community. Laura spends a lot of time with the people in her group home, so she enjoys getting away and doing something else. And mealtime seems just a good way to be together. —Rory Hoover, United States

At my group home, they follow the menu. I like everything. We eat at the dining room table, but one woman, she always acts up. She eats too fast and before dinner, she sometimes screams and cusses. I just eat and put the dishes in the dishwasher. I like getting out, especially when she says she's going to punch me. I used to work at the Burger King there on Federal behind the bushes, and they make me clean the men's toilet so I quit that job. —Laura Hinden, United States

Never talk past the person you are sharing mealtime with. Talk to that person. If you are talking with other people, too, make sure no one is left out. Explain what you're talking about, what the other person is saying, and involve them, even though the topic of conversation may not be fully understood by all.

Gone Fishing

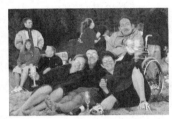

At the first light of the Millennium, January 1, 2000, Duncan, Julie, Mike, and Kaye share champagne on the beach.

We're a very outdoorsy family, and I don't know that we ever thought anything but doing whatever it took to make sure Duncan was there. We had the advantage of two older brothers, and Mike and Nigel were both big strong boys. But I was able to lift Duncan; Gary always said I had a neck and back like a weightlifter because as Duncan grew older and bigger, I just lifted more weight. I guess it's an attitude. Duncan was going to be with us. My dad built a little sedan chair with handles so we could carry Dunc down to the beach like an Egyptian pharaoh. We were all on the beach near Hawke's Bay to be the first to see the sunrise in 2000. We got about 3 or 4 hours of sleep and then we carried Duncan and hauled all of our beach stuff down to the beach at 5 A.M. and we all had our champers* to toast the New Millennium.

We always spent our holidays at my parents' beach house. My dad's fishing boat is just 12 feet long with a little outboard. We'd put Duncan in there and prop him up with lifejackets. He can hold the rod, and you don't have to cast for deep-sea fishing. He really enjoys those times. —Kaye Pollock, Australia

*champagne

Think of the person with a disability in terms of his or her chronological age as much as possible. Because helping someone eat is generally what we do with babies and young children, there is a danger of treating a person with a disability as an infant, stripping away self-esteem and falling prey to the old myth of the eternal child. Be sensitive.

Let Someone Else Be in Charge for a Change

As we've discussed, not everything has to be an educational or therapeutic experience. Sometimes individuals can derive great satisfaction from having control over their situations (see also Chapter 6). Bobo (Fred) Schwier, our son/brother Jim's grandfather, would agree:

> *I'll bet Jim would like to feel like he can really be the best at something, to do something real well—maybe even better than anyone else—for a change.*

Neil Mercer—who spent 13 years in an institution—suggests that an ideal home is more a state of being than a physical place or residential program. He doesn't talk about financial concerns or staff support. His first thought is of the kitchen and the fact he is both in charge and "a pretty darn good cook":

> *Someone once told me that a perfect home is where you can make yourself a bologna sandwich if you feel like it. And even better than that, you can wash it down with a beer if you want, and all in your underwear if you feel like it! The best thing I make is Mercer's Goulash. It's got hamburger and macaroni and some flour and mushrooms, if you like them, and pieces of onion. Then you put some spice in, but not that hot red stuff from Mexico! You can make it on the stove in a frying pan, in an electric pan, or even like a casserole in the oven. I sprinkle flour on top. I just made this recipe up and it's really good.*

 Think about what the home smells like. Are there institutional cleaners and odors, or are you welcomed with the aromas of baking, homemade dinner, and dessert in the oven?

Go Easy on the Advice

Parents whose children require various interventions sometimes feel overwhelmed with the opinions and suggestions from doctors, physical and occupational therapists, dieticians, and any number of health care professionals. Sometimes parents feel as though 24 hours in a day isn't half the time required to carry out all of these professionals' recommendations issued with the intent to help their child.

Families are feeling more empowered these days to say, "Enough is enough" when it comes to all of the professional intervention, however necessary and well intentioned, in their lives. In the Katoomba area of the Blue Mountains, New South Wales, Australian Goomblar Wylo says his son, Murrandah, has been "poked and prodded" by medical professionals from all over the world. Murrandah has both the rare Kabuki syndrome and Opitz syndrome. According to his family, he is the only documented person in the world known to have both. Goomblar says:

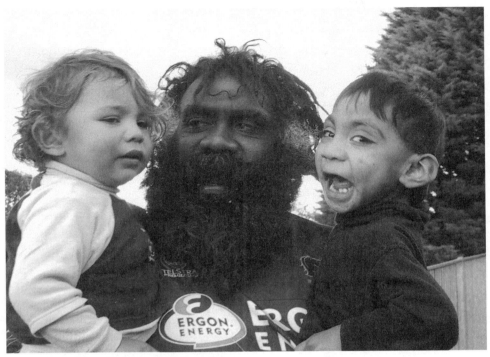

Burung, Goomblar, and Murrandah, Australia.

They come from all over to study him. Course, everybody wants to have a look. One time we were on holidays in Brisbane and he got sick. It's always a nightmare explaining to the doctors about Murrandah and what he has. When we'd go to the hospital, we'd get a lot of students, and a doctor would come in and say to the students, "So, what's wrong with the child?" They'd all talk about what's wrong with him, and there's poor wee Murrandah sitting on the bed. Then they'd want permission to photograph the boy. Then they'd want to take a bit of blood to study. He hates doctors, and as soon as one walks in the room his levels go up and the machines start beeping. Every doctor and their dog wants to come in and have a poke. Sometimes Murrandah isn't happy about it, and sometimes we say, "Right, mate, that's it. Piss off."

On the other end of the world, in northern Saskatchewan, Canada, Danny and Virginia Johns share Goomblar's sentiments. Their daughter, Wapunoohtiw, has De Soto syndrome. Their early childhood interventionist, Debra Menz, recalls leaving yet another medical appointment with the couple.

> As Danny stood with his wife and daughter in the hospital parking lot, he said they appreciated what everyone was trying to do. He said, "But we just want to be with our little girl. We just want to be a family and not worry about referrals and checklists for awhile." (Melberg Schwier, 20002001, p. 16)

It's important for families—and other caregivers—to remember that the advice of many practitioners is just that: advice. It's important to work with doctors and therapists as partners; your responsibility is to let them know what your lifestyle is like, and how and when your family will accommodate what is necessary.

Also remember that professionals aren't out to simply add more work, so helping them understand what and how therapies for the child and other arrangements can work best for your family is helpful. Some things aren't easily negotiable. Courses of medication, exercises, prohibitions on foods that may be harmful, or devices or practices to ensure personal health and safety are aspects of diagnosis and recommended amelioration that may not be open to much negotiation. Still, some day-to-day routines can be substituted for formal therapies.

The beauty of mealtime is that while it has therapeutic benefits in many ways, it doesn't have to be a "special" activity for people with disabilities that make them feel nothing but "disabled." It's just part of regular life, a social equalizer that presents opportunities to hang out and be regular. Perhaps a walk to a restaurant for dinner with friends once a week can replace the day's exercises. Spending an hour with a neighbor over lunch trying a delicious new finger food just might take the place of fine motor therapy now and then. Speech therapy might be the natural offshoot of a visit to the farmer's market when asking the vendors about their fruits, vegetables, and crafts. Many different solutions can fit various lifestyles in a better way.

 The Dining with Dignity program at Holy Name Hospital, Teaneck, New Jersey, was established by the Dysphagia Interdisciplinary Committee with the Food and Nutrition Services Department. There's a mouthful. With great success, they began serving puréed food that is reshaped to look like the real thing. Gelled cookies and carrot "coins" offer visual stimulation and texture to make eating more pleasurable.

Feel-Good Services

Services can be designed for people with disabilities that "feel right" and make people feel at home. Some of the homey atmosphere comes from attention to the table. One example is a long-term residential care home in San Diego, California, for children who have severe physical and intellectual disabilities who have become wards of the state. The home is operated by a couple who decided to open up their home after their retirement to no more than four children at a time; they were determined to make it feel like family. The house looked like any other in the neighborhood. Dorrie and Richard were about as much like "Mom and Dad" as anybody could be. The children living there were responsible for family chores and routines, so it just felt good

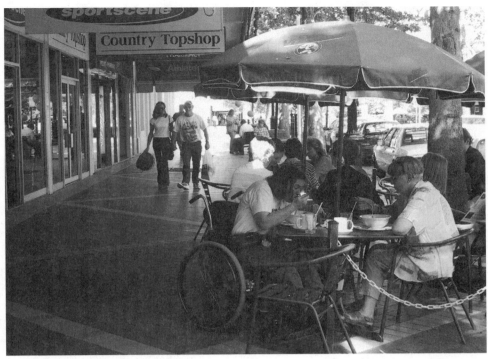

Check ahead to make sure the café or restaurant you choose is accessible. If the building itself isn't, and you're open to outdoor dining, you may still wish to patronize the place.

to be there. Erin (one of the authors) spent time there as a Resident Care Assistant while she attended college:

One Big Happy Family

I would be there when the bus brought the kids home from school. We would all have a snack, do homework, some therapy home program stuff, and play as Dorrie started dinner. We would all eat dinner together. All of the children needed extra help so each of us would help a child and eat our own dinner at the same time. A lot of attention was given to the favorite foods of each child. During dinner, we'd talk about school, things going on. We'd give opportunities for choice in what they were to eat next or help in their attempts to eat unassisted. After dinner it was bath time and quiet time. We read stories and the kids could watch favorite videos or the household favorite, *Wheel of Fortune,* before it was time for bed. When any of the kids had Open House at their schools, Dorrie and Richard would go. Richard built modified skateboards for some kids and on the weekends, we would take trips to the park to play. Hugs were given freely and smiles were encouraged. It was a great place to work; it didn't feel like work. I felt I had a family even though I was in college and away from my own.—Erin Schwier Stewart, United States

Children with disabilities need support to go through the messy developmental stage of exploring taste, texture, early grasp, and control of their environment. Sometimes older people with disabilities have missed this opportunity for discovery. We say better late than never! Put down a sheet for a picnic. Let everyone get messy. Encourage an older person with a disability to explore what food feels like, tastes like, how funny it can be when you throw it. No one should go through life without at least one food fight.

Forty-four-year-old Angela Fitzgerald was 10 when she was placed in a Canadian institution where she lived for 25 years. In the institutional setting, a suctioning machine was always nearby. Staff often strapped Angela—a tall, thin woman—into a chair to manage the speed with which she ate meals. Angela ate so rapidly that she often aspirated and had to be suctioned or even rushed to the hospital. On more than one occasion, her mother, Anne, was devastated by the advice of doctors to "just let her go." One nurse asked point-blank, "What kind of life can she possibly have anyway?" One day, Anne squared her shoulders, took a deep breath, and insisted it was not the life her daughter deserved.

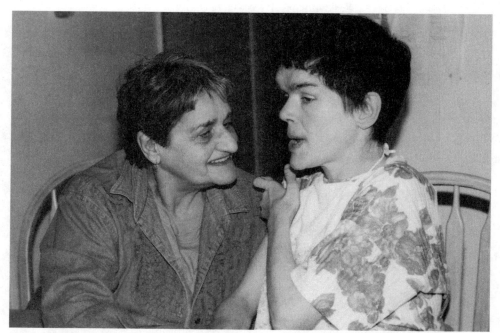

Anne and Angela Fitzgerald talk about the evening meal, taking some time to prepare and anticipate the food.

Anne felt that Angela, who was weakened from little activity, significant disabilities, and the repeated near-death bouts caused by inhaling food—including one that resulted in a collapsed lung—would indeed die unless she moved. Once she settled into a small group home, gentle, patient people surrounded Angela. They knew her old speed-eating habits would take a long time to fade. But fade they did during calm, soothing mealtimes where people offered Angela time and attention. "I think she started to feel safe and she knew she didn't have to eat so fast. She hasn't had to be suctioned once in that home and she even goes out to restaurants now," reports her mother. "I just can't believe the difference in her at mealtime. She enjoys her life and people enjoy her."

Hot dogs, candy, nuts, and grapes account for almost half of all choking deaths in young children (Harris, Baker, Smith, & Harris, 1984). Soft, loosely textured foods (such as bread) that become compressed upon swallowing are responsible for approximately 15% of such deaths (Dailey, 1983); this probably occurs more commonly in older children and adults with multiple disabilities. Danger foods can be ground and mixed with a little gravy. Without gravy or other moisture, ground food can often be sucked into the windpipe when breathing in. Grapes should be cut in half. There are companies that make puréed spread; you just add water and mix. Peanut butter, too, can be made edible by mixing in jelly or even soft tofu. Soft spreads such as marshmallow cream and peanut butter without jelly should be avoided (Sobsey & Thuppal, 1996).

If the person has significant disabilities, help her relax before mealtime begins. Talk about what you're doing, what you'll be eating, and when. Imagine what it might feel like to come to the table with tense muscles and no knowledge of what you'll be expected to eat.

Mealtime must be revered and taken seriously. If caregivers or family members find themselves in a position in which the dignity and respect of people is not being honored at mealtime, this situation should be questioned. Mealtime is a precious opportunity for communication and rich sensory experiences. If it's dismissed in 10 minutes to move on to other things such as (ironically) sensory stimulation therapy, we have to stand back and ask ourselves and others, "Why?"

If someone uses a tube at mealtime, the need for the mealtime experience still exists. Some people enjoy the sensory element of taste and enjoy something in their mouth. Some people are able to taste and spit; you can help this to happen discreetly.

 To share mealtimes with someone who makes use of a tube for food intake, learn a bit about this practice. There are nasogastric tubes (NG-tubes) that are inserted into one nostril, down the throat, and into the stomach. The stomach end has a rounded piece that allows liquid nourishment to flow into the stomach. Gastrostomy tubes (G-tubes) require surgical placement and deliver nourishment directly to the stomach. Remember that enjoyment of the mealtime experience is a lot more than just the insertion of nutrients!

 Always wash your hands carefully with soap and water before doing any care of someone's tube.

Lunch with the Guys

I go to lunch with some of the guys from the town work crew and we discuss things. I like to go to the bus depot for lunch. I eat grill ham and cheese or grill bacon and cheese. I watch to see they do a proper job, just melt the cheese in perfect. They don't like me watching over their shoulder! At the bus depot, there's a Chinese woman, she is real young, but she's a good cook. The reason I go there for lunch with the guys is that we chat about business and politics. That's mostly how it is. —James Necula, Canada

Dinner Conversation

We talk a lot about my upcoming wedding. I can't say Laura really confides her inner-most feelings to me. She's a private person, but we enjoy just talking about day-to-day things. I think Laura knows she can talk to me about anything. We have more of a companionable friendship. We yak. We catch up and fill each other in on our lives. And going out for lunch or dinner just seems to be a nice relaxed time for us. I remember the first time we went out for a meal at Burger King, she said my hair was beautiful. —Rory Hoover, United States

Sharing is nice. First time we got together, I said, "It's a match!" We talk about good times. Always talk about the wedding. She's marrying Bart Simpson. His name is Bart. Rory is moving away so instead of Best Buddies, we're gonna be Pen Pals. I'll get another Best Buddy. We like to go eat. We went to Moe's restaurant, and it was strange. The menu was on the wall and we had to look on the wall to order. My favorite is Mexican. We went to the Miami Seaquarium. Had soy burger. That wasn't good. I like the greater outdoors. —Laura Hinden, United States

Consider what you have in common with the person you are dining with in addition to the food you are eating. This can make for better mealtime conversation. Are you both Trekkies? Maybe you've been to the same places.

See People as People, Vices and All

Similar to the opinion that all activities have to be special or therapeutic is the idea some people have that people with disabilities can't or shouldn't enjoy the same recreational pastimes surrounding food and drink that everyone else does. Some believe that everything eaten or imbibed has to be healthy. Although well-intentioned, today we realize that true inclusion means that people have the right to relax and enjoy the same things everyone else does, such as an alcoholic beverage (assuming that they're of legal drinking age and it wouldn't be harmful to their health or condition).

Show Off Some Skills

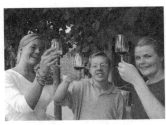

Jim shares a toast with travelers.

Because he helps his father to make wine at home in the basement, Jim knows to hold a small sample up to the light to gaze knowingly at the color and make the appropriate remarks. At a tasting at the Tulloch Winery in Australia's Hunter Valley, Jim demonstrates the technique to Ingunn Starem and Susanne Hjorth Blystad, two traveling Norwegians. "He really knows a lot about the wine!" Ingunn says. Swirling the wine in the glass is known as *volatizing the esters*. This releases the wine's aromas. Inhale over the rim of the glass and try to put a name to it—oak, peppery, black currant? The smell of the wine is its *nose*. Take a mouthful and swish it around. Choose to swallow, or spit like the professionals. This lesson can be pared down to, "Hold it up. Look at light. Smell it. Taste it." Any way you choose, a little vintner knowledge is very impressive! —Karin Melberg Schwier, Canada

Just Another Bloke

Stan enjoyed going to the movies. Every Saturday night. In those days you could take food in, not like the posh theatres now where you can't bring in your own tucker*. They used to let you take the lot in. And what's more, they had fellas selling. It was open slather**, anything you wanted. There was a meat pie man, a bloke selling hot dogs. Stan used to get himself a meat pie for the movie. He thought that was a real go. And he enjoyed his beer, Stan did. Once he was staying with my sister; she had a hotel. She called me. "Quick," she says, "Stan's had a stroke." I said, "I dunno. Are you sure?" She'd given Stan six cans of beer so he could have a shandy*** every day for a week. I said, "I reckon he's drunk." "No, no, can't be," she said. "He's only had one can. All the rest are in the fridge." Well, it was a stinkin' hot day and he was clever, old Stan. He'd put the little tabs back on and put the empties back in the fridge. He was short, but he was a stocky bloke. Still, he wasn't used to having more than one. Toohey's Flag it was, blue cans. Shocking drunk, he was. —Rod Hall, Australia

 *Food
 **A large variety of food choices
***Beer and lemonade

Things are Cooking Up

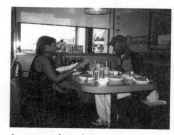

Aunya and Carl meet sometimes for breakfast and catch up on each other's lives.

Something we haven't done together yet is cook. I'm from New Orleans, so everyone in my family cooks and it's hard for me to cook for just one. But sometimes I get in the mood to fix fish, some kind of meat. I use a lot of ground turkey. There's usually a New Orleans twist to it; people would recognize the spice! I'm the breakfast girl in the family; my sister does dinner. I like to make omelettes, biscuits, pancakes. I'll make it all for the same meal. I think it's something fun Carl and I could do together. —Aunya Honore, United States

I cook breakfast. You know, I cook in my parents' house, like fried chicken, chicken wings, and that; when I went to the group home, I cook eggs right now and bacon. I make pancakes. You know, you just read the directions on the box and mix it all right up. I make good pancakes and I'm gonna get a moped but I be real careful so I don't get into no accident. I'm gonna do more cookin' when I am not studying for my license. Maybe Aunya and me, we make a pizza. We could make that. She don't like no blue cheese, but anyways, I just have blue cheese on my half of the pizza we make. Blue cheese, it is stayin' on my half, okay? That'd be delicious for me. And then I get my license. —Carl Shell, United States

Restaurant Routine

Back then, Boggabri wasn't very big so we used to go into Gunnedah, the next town, every Friday to do the shopping and then stop in at the Acropolis for a meal. Stan used to have the same meal every time. He'd buy batteries for his little radio and he'd buy razorblades whether he needed them or not. And then he'd have the sausage and eggs. He could have had anything, but he thought that was the go. Best thing on the menu. A bit of grilled tomato. That was a bit of all right, sausage and eggs every Friday at the Acropolis with Mum and Dad. —Rod Hall, Australia

 For some people, mealtime may be the best chance during the day to spend time with someone who will focus on them completely.

SHAKE WHAT YOU'VE GOT, "CULINARILY" SPEAKING

Showing off a little can be a powerful social tool to initiate membership. When you think about it, interesting people have done and can talk about lots of things, and they're willing and able to listen to us talk about what we know. If people cannot tell their own stories, others can do so for them. We belong when others want us to belong. Some interesting tidbits of information or skills help with the small talk at mealtimes, for example, making us just a little bit more desirable to the group. We can work at becoming a member of one group or another, but our entry ultimately depends on how well we are able to influence what the group decides.

Friends, family, and caregivers who know a person with a disability well can elevate the expectations and impressions others have of the individual. By adding elements that are valued in our society, we take advantage of the multiplier effect. Someone with a noticeable disability who is sociable and friendly is more accepted in our culture, more likely to be liked by others. If he is sociable, friendly, *and* dresses and grooms well, even better. In addition, if an individual is in possession of a skill or item that is highly valued, people are even more impressed. As we raise the expectations of others toward people with disabilities, we open the door to potential connections. People with disabilities can help others realize that they have something to contribute to the community and help them understand that they are here to give back, not just to receive. Real membership and participation in community is based on that give and take.

Robyn Hadfield speaks of her parents' expectations for all of her siblings, not just for her sister, Dorothy, who has Down syndrome. While she's not certain that her par-

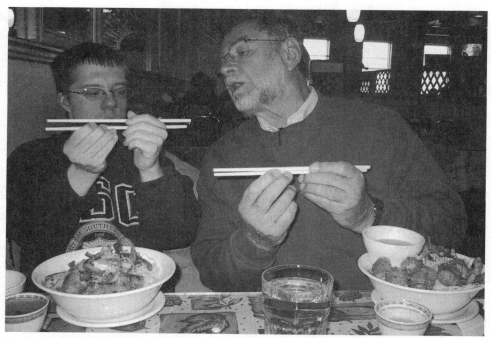

Jim (left), an adept chopstick user, gives Robert some tips on how to hold them. It didn't help; Robert enjoyed his chicken saté with a fork.

ents intentionally gave Dorothy responsibilities in order to help her develop a strong sense of self-esteem, she does know that her sister's sense of self-worth as an adult is solid:

> I can't remember a time when Dorothy didn't set the table, set things out, wash up, wipe up. I think she likes to do those things because she knows what to do and that makes her feel good. Mum, Dad, and Dorothy are all creatures of habit and so they eat at approximately the same time each day. Dorothy knows what to do and can anticipate. In fact, she would anticipate Dad wanting a cup of tea so she'd go make him one and one for Mum as well. She'll shell the peas that Dad's got out of the garden, peel the vegetables, things like that. I don't think Dorothy would ever be able to just sit there without getting up to help. There were chores all of us were expected to do, so Dorothy was no different.

Show Me How Much

Some people require more structure, more detail. I talk to one woman who wants to know how I cook something and I say, "Oh, I just throw some of this and put some of that" and she says, "No, I need to know exactly how much!" This is true for some people with disabilities. If they want to learn how to cook something, maybe you are more specific. Okay, you want to make the pasta. You have to take a pot. Which pot? This one, this big. You have to fill it with water, to here. Maybe you have to mark it on the pot. See, this much olive oil. Nothing can be taken for granted. With some people they learn if you break it into very small pieces. I think this is the way it is going to be for Andrea.—Edi Cicchini, Italy

Knowledge, skill, and an appreciation of mealtime are opportunities to contribute in ways others might not have expected. Bringing a chickpea salad (see recipe, p. 210) to the company potluck is impressive in the eyes of a co-worker. The "Wow, I didn't think you could make something like that!" response can have a big payoff, such as an invitation to the next block party. It may even plant the seed of a common topic of conversation. Knowing how to whip up some authentic Chinese fried cabbage (see recipe, p. 214) at home or being able to handle chopsticks in a restaurant can raise some eyebrows and expectations.

And there's nothing better than good gossip, especially if it's something good about the listener. Let someone with a disability overhear you saying great things about her contributions to the meal. These contributions can be big or small. Helping prepare the main course, setting the table, arranging the flowers, or even simply appreciating the wonderful smells in the kitchen are all valued ways to participate and interact. Culinary skills and the self-confidence they induce help to us leap ahead—or even take just a few steps—in the game of expectations.

Togetherness

When we go to Mum's now, we all involve Margie more. Come on, let's get the biscuits and cheese. You know where the biscuits are, could you get them for me please? Can you pour your orange juice? We're learning how to help Margie be a part of everything by helping her be a part of everything. She does often need assistance. For example, if there's a big bottle of orange juice, she can't pour it by herself, but if I help her hold it, she can pour it. We can do it together. —Beth Macleod, Australia

 Have trouble holding onto utensils? Velcro bands with a pocket at the palm of the hand (sometimes called a "universal cuff") can be used to insert a spoon or a fork and can be wrapped around a hand.

 Bendable utensils and jar and bottle openers make handling objects easier.

Some spoons have sharp edges. One of the best spoons for some people with disabilities is the type with a vinyl covering to avoid injury. White is the most common but tends to stain from tomato and curry sauces. Red is a little startling. Try navy blue. Avoid baby utensils; ask at a kitchen supply store if less-juvenile looking ones can be ordered.

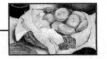

CHAPTER 5

Connecting with Catherine

SHERRILL RUCKERT

Catherine Schaefer has never been able to speak or walk. As a friend of her mother, Nicola Schaefer, I had seen her for many years, from a distance, at parties in their home. Catherine sits with support and needs total assistance. I seemed always to be present when some good-intentioned soul would feed her food she was unable to swallow and she would have what her mother called one of her "spectacular chokes" and need emergency response in the middle of the party. I tried to communicate with Catherine on several occasions, but she refused to make eye contact with me or brushed my hand away.

At the age of 25, Catherine moved into her own home. In cooperation with David Wetherow, the executive director for the Association for Community Living, Winnipeg Branch, Nicola set up a large, three-apartment house on the edge of Vimy Ridge Park in Winnipeg. Catherine shared the main floor apartment with another young woman who was her primary caregiver and managed the household and respite staff. From her new home, Catherine attended several day programs including those offered by a local high school, Gordon Bell; the University of Winnipeg; and Red River Community College.

I first saw Catherine living independently during a house blessing conducted for the new household and all of its occupants. After the blessing, we celebrated with a picnic in the park across the street. I was there that day with my three young children, Nicola, and David, who was then my husband. The warm camaraderie of the group and Catherine's sparkling, beautiful eyes were very inviting. I wondered what it would be like to be part of this small, created community with Catherine as the heart.

David and I separated years later, when my children ranged in age from 13 to 20 years old. After several years passed, I rented a large upstairs apartment in Nicola's house in River Heights, together with my two sons, Dante and Owen. An exchange

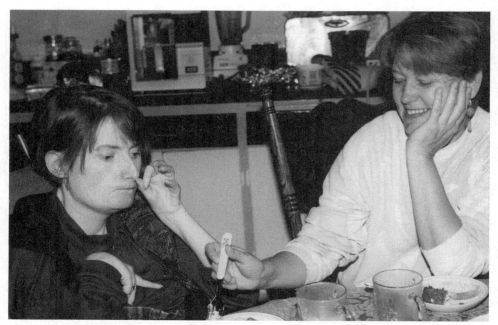

Catherine (left) and Sherrill share a relaxing meal.

student from Japan, Rhuji Shimoda, joined us. Nicola's half of the house was filled with visitors from around the world, many of them musicians or respite workers from the L'Arche Community. Catherine was also a visitor during family celebrations and holidays, sometimes for several weeks at a time. We shared many communal meals, which sometimes included my daughter, Alia, and her husband, Paul. On special occasions, Catherine's two brothers, Dominic and Ben, would join us for visits when they were in town. Catherine was always at the table with us, excited by all of the company, especially her brothers and the young men from my household. When I entertained in my place, they would carry her, fireman's style, up the long wide staircase and haul her elongated wheelchair up to seat her comfortably at the table. Catherine stayed the course at these times, obviously enjoying the stories and the food. Nicola usually shared her meal with her daughter, spoon and hand feeding her most things. Catherine would occasionally grab the spoon in frustration or snitch a piece of food from the plate with her working left hand if Nicola was too engaged by someone else. She could grasp a piece of bread and bring it to her mouth, although it sometimes dropped to the table or floor. Mechanics aside, Catherine relished the communal breaking of bread.

The ritual of eating was often a source of "heart to heart" connection between mother and daughter, embellished as it was by life's chatter, friends, music and Nicola's singing. Often while visiting in Nicola's kitchen, I ventured to assist Catherine in sipping her favorite cup of tea—Earl Grey—with lots of cream and sugar. English to the core, like her mother.

One day, while I was visiting her mother, I was asked to sit with Catherine while Nicola went out for the evening. I had just completed a course in Reiki, a form of hands-on energy work. So as we sat watching television together, I placed my hand on Catherine tentatively, sending her energy. She didn't brush me away this time. In fact, after about 20 minutes of this kind of touch, she made clear eye contact. I moved my hand to another location and again was accepted. Nicola had written a book about Catherine titled *Does She Know She's Here?,* and I had always been curious to know Catherine for myself. I told Nicola about our evening when she returned, and Nicola hired me to visit regularly with Catherine, who was then already living in her own home with 24-hour support. Over time I extended my contact to foot and back massage and eventually volunteered to live as Catherine's primary caregiver when the current one became ill.

I had been renting my apartment for nearly 2 years at that time, and my sons and Rhuji were ready to move on with their lives. The apartment was too large for one person and Catherine's house was only a few blocks from Manitoba Education where I worked as the coordinator for Braille production. It was a challenging order to live in with Catherine, running her household while continuing with outside full-time employment, but I like challenges. The salary of a live-in primary caregiver would be too meager to pay my bills, so I chose to do both with the support of respite staff.

Catherine had then been living in her house for 10 years, so we planned a large anniversary party and invited all of those who had lived with her over the years as well as family and friends. In preparation for that celebration, I hired a friend to assist me in sprucing up the grounds and our apartment, which were showing some signs of their age. I supervised these activities before moving in and concentrated on Catherine once I was there. We began with some attention to her hair and wardrobe, having great fun together shopping at the local Value Village for new clothes after having her "colors" done. I would hold up an item that was in her color and size range, and Catherine would indicate with hand or facial gestures whether it met her approval. She and her wheelchair soon disappeared beneath a huge stack of accepted articles of clothing. Catherine's family had supplied her with an adapted van, so we were able to travel together for shopping, movies, adventures out of the city, and many more within. So we began this leg of our journey together, once again with friends, music, stories, flowers from our garden and Nicola's, and, of course a potluck menu contributed to by all. Because it was also Catherine's birthday, there were wonderful gifts from those who knew her well and who had cherished her for many years. We were off to a good start.

Over the 2½ years I lived with her, I came to know that Cath is indeed here; more present actually than many people I have known who walk and talk quite regularly. For myself, I learned that speech is not necessary for intimacy. The presence of the other is all that is truly required. Catherine had much physical suffering to endure at times as well as all of the limitations in movement and speech, yet she was able to be joyful, humorous, sad, and grateful, and she communicated and shared daily life with me.

Cath seemed to enjoy eating during simple social interaction more than at any other time. She regulates her own diet with awareness that many would envy. She maintains a perfect weight for herself, eating only what she wants, when she wants it. She enjoys meat, fish, and poultry of many kinds as long as it is moist and cut into reasonably sized pieces. Like many people with cerebral palsy-like conditions, she doesn't chew her food very well. Potatoes, rice, and vegetables also need to be moist and easy to swallow. Things such as nuts, raw carrots and celery, crackers, popcorn, hard candies, and even peanut butter can create real hazards from choking and aspirating into her lungs. A few years before I began living with Cath, she was found to have a huge hiatal hernia complicated by large cysts on her ovaries. Before these conditions were corrected surgically, she was often in pain from the searing stomach acid that badly scarred her esophagus and the pneumonia that often followed aspirating food. Repeated bouts of pneumonia necessitated antibiotic regimes that left her with yeast and bladder infections in their wake. I noticed that Catherine showed an aversion to acidic foods such as vinegar, orange juice, and heavy tomato sauces, so I eliminated them from her diet. I served her salads with lots of creamy dressing or a homemade lemon juice and olive oil with herbs. Baked apples instead of raw ones, ripe pears, berries, and bananas were favorites. I selected moist whole-grain breads. Toast was always lightly done and moistened with a generous amount of butter and olive oil. Yogurt was a staple that helped normalize her intestinal flora. She preferred it with fruit and/or honey.

Cath loved her coffee and her tea, but I was concerned that too much caffeine stimulation for a person who took medication for seizure activity was unwise. In addition, because of lack of physical exercise, keeping her bowels moving was a concern. Because both coffee and tea are diuretics as well as quite acidic, I looked for another source of warm drinks that would be popular with her. Cath wasn't particularly fond of herbal teas (I later discovered that peppermint tea causes the sphincter muscle of the esophagus to relax and can encourage reflux for those who are susceptible). Fortunately, I discovered a product that fit the bill, a coffee substitute, Inka. Served with milk and honey, it helped keep her hydrated and provided a mild stimulation to her bowels. Best of all, she really enjoyed her new "cuppa," and she sipped a cup throughout the day, including her times at the day program.

To her basically good diet I added high-quality vitamins, which included evening primrose oil (for better neural transmission) and a buffered vitamin C. Given with her morning and evening medication, they were washed down with a warm cup of Inka after being placed at the back of her throat for ease in swallowing.

In periods of illness, Cath usually stopped eating, so the Inka became an important source of both water and food during such times. Drinking and sleeping freely helped her heal quickly from most common colds and viruses, often more quickly than those around her. During one more lengthy illness I made a "miracle" discovery with the aid of a slow cooker. I put chicken bones in the pot with a few tablespoons of vinegar to soften them and leach the calcium into the broth. To the broth I added 30 cloves of garlic, carrots and/or yams, and some chicken pieces. After slow cooking this mixture overnight, I puréed all the ingredients, including the soft bones. Catherine ate seven bowls and quickly regained her strength. Generally, however, puréed foods were unnecessary. She did sometimes enjoy nutritious fruit smoothies, but more often preferred "regular people food." Like most people, she especially enjoyed her mother's English-style cooking, and she usually increased her food intake during home visits.

Some of the respite workers enjoyed baking with Catherine. She often had a hand in the cookie pressing or in tasting the dough. Homemade muffins and cookies with Inka helped round out the menu for afternoon tea. On mornings when Handi-Transit arrived far ahead of schedule, we would include a muffin and yogurt in her lunch box to fill the gap. Bananas were a standby when time was limited. Easy to transport, chew, and digest, they also helped absorb the stomach acid that continues to be an issue. I did eventually convince her doctor to give her a prescription antacid that helped her to stay more comfortable.

To facilitate continuity in her care, we maintained a small daily diary that noted her food intake, behavior, moods, and any onset of illness or indication of pain. The diary traveled with her wherever she went and provided an invaluable source of information for new staff and even for her mother when she would return home for visits. All staff were free to include any anecdotes from the day as well as to note the more mundane losses of hairbrushes, lunch kits, and so forth, so it became a great way also to include conversation about her day with Cath over the evening meal.

Sunday morning was often special for us; the slow pace was possible because both of us were home for the day. Sunday breakfast was usually in bed as we both enjoyed sleeping in a bit. I had bought Cath a festive kimono for occasions like this, so I'd begin by draping it over her shoulders and opening the curtains before bringing in a tray with a hot breakfast for both of us. I offered any combination of whole-grain pancakes with maple syrup, soft-boiled eggs, yogurt and banana, or possibly just toast and Inka if she was eating lightly. The casual pleasure of such Sunday mornings was in strong contrast to the necessary rush of weekdays when Cath needed to be ready for Handi-Transit to take her to her day program. But on Sundays, she often greeted me with hoots and giggles, knowing the morning would be enjoyable. Hair washing, a massage, and a long soak in the jacuzzi would follow this leisurely breakfast. My singing and chanting always punctuated her lovely water stretches. Her first recognized word, "home," had its beginning in the Ohm I chanted in the jacuzzi while placing my hands on her diaphragm and lower back.

Another favorite was having guests for dinner. Cath usually grinned when I announced the coming of certain guests, preferably male. She would often feed herself more independently in the presence of guests and particularly enjoyed lingering over a meal for long periods filled with conversation. Much as she was unable to verbalize herself, Cath enjoyed listening to words being spoken, whether in conversation or read aloud from a book. Although I often chattered on as we carried out the daily activities, conversation between two people seemed considerably more interesting to her. Family meals to which I would invite my adult children were another favorite. During these times she would want to try what everyone else was eating and would snatch a favorite item off the plate of someone seated beside her. We would always remove the tray from her chair so she could sit up to the table with the rest of us. Cath seemed to be very amused with family-type interactions and responded with big smiles to the attention of my two sons. I suspect that these meals mirrored her childhood family times when she had the attention of her two brothers.

I always enjoyed going out to dinner with Cath. It was a chance to connect with each other without all the fuss of meal preparation. Sharing a meal with lots of time to taste and comment seemed to perk Cath's appetite as well as mine. In the good weather, we would visit local establishments, enjoying a walk through the neighboring streets and parks as part of our outing. When I had help, we would picnic in the park across the street on a blanket. She enjoyed being down on the ground with a large body pillow for support, but it took at least two people to lift her up and down from her wheelchair. When this wasn't possible, I would share snacks with her sitting beside a park bench and watch the young neighborhood children at play on the swings and waterslide. During the summer months, musicians often performed in the park, creating wonderful, inexpensive entertainment. At times, a walk across the main street to McDonald's for an order of fries was just to her taste. We traveled about the city in her van visiting a wide variety of restaurants. To minimize costs I would place a single order with perhaps a side dish and we would share it. Restaurant staff were usually helpful in making room for her large chair, though some restaurants were a little difficult to enter. Popular nearby Corydon Avenue, with outdoor seating, has great places to hang out while enjoying some gelati or a full-course meal. Catherine really enjoyed people watching, especially handsome young men.

In the summer months we also ventured into the outlying provincial parks and beaches. Picnic tables were always accessible, and she loved swimming when the water was warm enough. I attempted beach outings on my own a few times and even purchased a wetsuit for Catherine for colder waters, but struggling with the wheelchair and lifting on the sand was a bit too much. Whenever possible I learned to invite others who could help or hired respite staff to accompany us.

Some of the other staff—those who were not living in the household—really enjoyed sharing the preparation of a meal with Cath. Being included meant being able to make choices before dinner as well as during. We tried creating a basic menu book with photographs, hoping that Cath would indicate her choices by pointing. This didn't work; however, she would point to items she wanted if they were put in front of her. There were many reports of Cath's excitement over foods she had watched being prepared, but she would still refuse anything hands down if she didn't like or want it after it was actually prepared. Social placating is not one of her traits.

For several summers, Cath and I would join my partner, Don, at our summer cottage on the lake. Cath enjoyed the barbecues and sing-alongs with the neighbors, visits from friends with backyard picnics, and trips to some of the favorite local eating spots. Although I was often busy with entertaining, there was always someone to share food with Cath. People just getting to know her sensed that sharing food might be a way to begin a connection. I usually started them off helping her with a beverage. When they appeared comfortable, I brought pre-selected foods for them to offer or placed items on her wheelchair tray that she could handle herself. We installed a new tray with a raised lip that kept food from falling and provided an edge she could use to help keep food in place while she was grasping it. The tray was made of molded heavy-duty plastic that was easy to keep clean. Also transparent, it allowed Cath to see her own legs and feet.

The size of the gathering seemed to be a factor in Cath's appetite. As long as the number of partygoers was reasonable and the noise low, she showed a strong interest and pleasure in sharing the spread. I noticed, however, that at large and noisy parties, she often showed little interest. It was as though too much stimulation just took her appetite away. She would also grow tired easily in this type of situation and probably enjoyed prepping for the party more than actually being there. With a new outfit and hairdo, Cath would light up at the positive comments on her appearance made by friends and family.

Most important is to emphasize the pleasure that sharing a meal brings. Eating with Cath rather than feeding her increased our communication and probably enhanced nutrition as well. Because of her physical vulnerability and the number of people involved in her care, there is always a keen awareness of her health and diet. At times this helped create an atmosphere of anxiety about both the quality and quantity of her food and liquid intake. When such concerns began to take precedence over simply enjoying Catherine's presence, I noticed she would withdraw into herself, not really wanting to eat or drink. Making mealtimes special again in the ways I've described was the most important ingredient in the return of her good appetite.

After Catherine left her family home, her new caregivers worked diligently to help her eat more independently. She was encouraged to use a specially designed spoon and her food was placed in a bowl on a sticky mat to keep it from sliding. In times of high energy, Cath enjoyed using her new skill; however, it could become laborious. Unfortunately, feeding herself could also add to social isolation. Whereas others can command attention through speech, even across a room, she needed closer contact to connect. I learned to appreciate the closeness that sharing food brings as more important than how independent Catherine could become. She grew up in a sociable and very loving family that prized the sharing of food together. Now in her adult living situation, where frequently changing staff members replace the care of family members, breaking bread together has become an even more important avenue for turning strangers into friends. Nothing lubricates the digestive system like enjoying yourself and others. This is the daily communion that is so important to share.

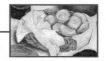

CHAPTER 6

The Hunger for Choice and Control

*Part of the secret in life is to eat
what you like and let the food fight it out on the inside.*
—MARK TWAIN (AS CITED IN FERRER, 2004)

If choice and variety weren't such important elements in food consumption, then restaurants would have a much simpler time. They could dispense with menus and offer one item, prepared one way, day after day. Beef lasagna, that's it. Broiled fish, stir-fry veggies, and new potatoes? Don't think so. But a restaurant with such an attitude would be out of business in a week. Even cafés specializing in one type of thing, such as soup, often have a range of choices and typically a few add-ons as well. The Scandinavians got it right when they invented the smörgåsbord. People like to have their favorites, but also they want the power and freedom to make choices and experiment.

Yet, for many people with disabilities, opportunities to have choice, variety, and even a chance to eat outside a schedule are absent or, at best, fleeting. Agency routine and concerns that "It'll take too long," or "This is the way we've always done it" too often dictate the interactions between caregivers and people with disabilities. Yet, one study (Reid & Parsons, 1991) found that when caregivers who served people with disabilities lunch each day were trained to offer more choices during the meal (e.g., fries with or without ketchup, more of the same beverage or something different), the mealtimes were lengthened by only a few minutes in the process. So the old "It'll be faster if I just do it myself" lament of staff who balk at the idea of introducing choice making to mealtimes hasn't much foundation.

Mealtime is a rich and renewable learning opportunity. Because so many activities and tasks are associated with it, children with disabilities can exercise their decision-making powers and their growing sense of self by participating in many ways. It may sound silly to connect the act of deciding that "The blue napkins will go on the table instead of the yellow ones Mom suggested" to the ability to make more serious life decisions later on. But starting small and working up is often a successful approach to building self-confidence.

Learning as a child to say no and to be heard plants the seeds of legitimate self-protection in adolescence and adulthood. So beginning in toddlerhood, children need to be offered choices, and their choices need to be respected. It's actually fairly easy to teach choice making. Part of this process is teaching someone to indicate when his or her choice *isn't* honored.

> Imagine asking your child if he wants corn or peas. If he says, "Corn, please," you say, "Okay, we'll do it your way. Peas it is." If your child doesn't kick up a fuss, you have some work to do. You want your child to say, in some form, "Hey, I said I wanted corn." (Melberg Schwier & Hingsburger, 2000, p. 145)

Mealtimes typically provide numerous opportunities, both verbal and nonverbal, for an individual to make sure that his or her wishes have been heard and to make sure that they are respected. In order for choices to be made, they must be heard and action taken to honor them. Mealtime choice making is a skill developed over time, as families teach and expect children to take on additional responsibilities while they learn and grow. The issue of choice can be tricky. "How much," "what," and "when" to eat or have a mealtime varies widely from family to family and in different situations. It doesn't mean you relinquish all the decision-making to your child. Try to think more in terms of supported decision-making. One parent, D. West, looks at it this way:

> *Because my child has an [intellectual] disability, we have to help him with the choices he makes and still try to get him to think about consequences of doing one thing or another. At this point, if we turned over the decision-making to him, he'd choose a large bowl of ice cream and M&Ms in front of the TV for every meal. Are we infringing on his right to choice by saying "No, you aren't going to do that"? I don't think we are.*

A CHOICE ISN'T A CHOICE UNLESS IT'S REAL

Choices should be real. A multiple choice between two or three things a person doesn't like or want isn't a choice at all. To offer someone who doesn't like vegetables a "choice" between broccoli or asparagus is not helping her understand that choice can mean being able to say "No, thanks." Of course, there are times when parents and caregivers aren't really prepared to accept a particular choice. Part of being in a family means compromise and learning to experience and enjoy new things. But a choice shouldn't be offered if you have no intention of following through. As an individual

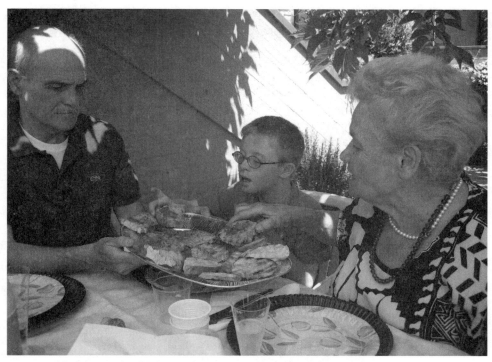

Ten-year-old Andrea makes his own selection as a plate of bruschetta is offered.

grows, families and caregivers must adjust their views to ensure that real choice is supported and respected if the person is to be seen as a whole human being with his own legitimate opinions and desires.

 Remember that someone may have had a "bad food experience" in the past. Perhaps they were forced to eat something they didn't like. Don't force people to eat something.

 Is the food being served to someone with a disability something you would enjoy or would just tolerate?

 Add color to meals. Cauliflower, mashed potatoes, and steamed whitefish might be nutritious, but how blah they look! Color stimulates interest and visual enjoyment of foods.

Leigh Chou's son, Daniel, has autism and some accompanying issues around food tolerance. Even with Daniel's food restrictions, Leigh is prepared to allow some flexibility from time to time in order to support Daniel's growing sense of exploration and independence:

> *At Red Lobster once, he reached over and grabbed a fried shrimp off of my plate. He didn't mind the touch and nibbled all the breading off of it like a tiny corncob. We knew he shouldn't have the bread, but we were so curious about what he was doing and that he was trying something new. Sometimes you've just got to let him be in charge a little bit.*

Dr. Stephanie Baars is an occupational therapist in Los Angeles, California, who believes that making choices builds a sense of autonomy. She promotes occupational self-analysis based on the concept of "lifestyle redesign," originated by Dr. Florence Clark in the University of Southern California's Well Elderly Study. Empowering people with disabilities to make choices on a regular basis is even more important because, Baars says:

> *Habits like taking initiative, thinking for oneself, and becoming comfortable with daily routines can take some consistent support to be sure they take hold in someone's repertoire of abilities. Habits and routines are extremely important to develop because they really make life easier.*
>
> *Can you imagine having to think of everything that you need to do each day like it was the first time you ever tried it? Take your morning routine, for example. I get up, go to the bathroom, brush my teeth and then get in the shower. Without fail. I even have a routine in the shower that seldom changes. By having routines and habits in our days, we have more time and energy to devote to other new and challenging activities.*

Developing mealtime habits, too, offers opportunities for small responsibilities and choices that become comfortably familiar and that can grow over time. Children learn to set the table, even if it just starts with getting the napkins to the dining room. Getting the pickle dish ready, arranging the rolls on a plate, and filling the water glasses all are empowering activities that make the child part of the social activity of family mealtime. As each small task becomes a familiar habit, choices and decisions about other activities are added. Grocery shopping, gardening, pick-your-own produce outings, visits to the farmer's market, and cooking are all tasks that encourage decision-making, choice, communication, and self-confidence.

 Everyone likes to go places where people know their name. Get to know local shopkeepers. Model friendly and courteous behavior. Always involve the person with the disability in the exchange, whether it's a chat in the aisle or making the purchases at the register.

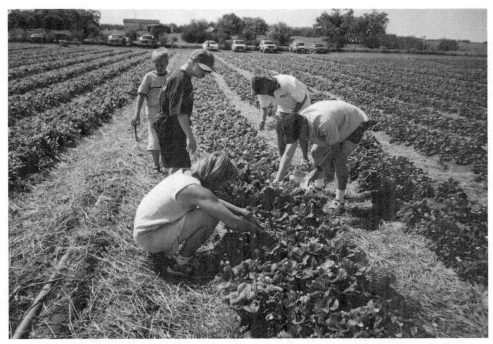

"Pick-your-own" outings are great for friends and family, and the bounty offers opportunities for canning and freezing.

 Investigate neighborhood teas and potlucks. They're a great opportunity for getting to know the neighbors and an excuse to get cooking.

Part of supporting choice-making skills means getting to know someone's learning styles, says Baars. Does the person respond more to visual, auditory, or kinesthetic cues? Perhaps a combination of these works well for the individual. Does the person respond better to pictures of the type of food she might choose at the grocery or is she better able to help with cooking when recipes are illustrated?

If you determine that the person responds well to spoken instructions, breaking down the steps and explaining each one might be helpful. Begin with tackling the first or last step (forward or backward chaining) and go from there. Some people need to try things for themselves several times over until they understand. "There have been plenty of work-site studies that show that increased involvement in the decision-making process is correlated with higher levels of satisfaction," says Baars. "I think this holds true in any situation. People want to feel like they have control in what they do each day. They will feel more invested in the situation and will work harder to make sure they succeed."

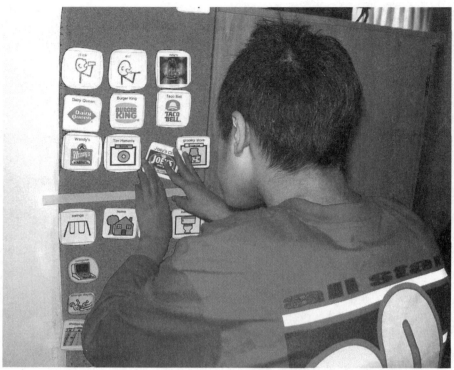

David decides on Joey's Seafood as the place to be for dinner. David is supported to make thoughtful decisions and express choices with symbols he can peel off and present to his family.

Here is a great tip for people who use Velcro symbols. Try a wall-mounted communication board made up of a 2-foot by 2-foot carpet runner. You can get one at Home Depot for about $4. It's glued to the wall with contact cement and various symbols, like which restaurant sounds good for supper, and can be backed with Velcro and peeled off the board when it's time to make a choice.

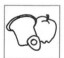

Offer choices about when to eat, how the table might be decorated, and if the meal should be served up at the stove or family-style at the table.

I'm Ready Now

Andrea refused to chew until just recently, and he is 10 years old. He was eating homogenized food, and we gradually started to increase the texture so that he could feel something in his mouth. But he still would not chew, no attempt to chew, just to swallow. No interest in trying new things. You know how small children will play with their food and try little tastes of things. Other kids, they like chocolate and things like that. But not Andrea, nothing. At school he would be having his lunch, and they tried all sorts of strategies and they just ended up with homogenized. He just did not like to put things in his mouth. At first it was difficult with tooth brushing and splashing the water, but he has overcome this. But food, this was a different matter. Then one day, his teacher came straight out of the school to me and she say, 'I have to tell you, Andrea has been biting.' And I thought, 'Oh no! Not a child. Oh, no!' She said, 'No, don't worry, it is only a tortellino!' —Edi Cecchini, Italy

GAINING SOME CALORIE CONTROL

How do you help someone with an intellectual disability grasp a concept as complex as lowering caloric and fat intake in order to lose weight? How do you impress upon anybody that maintaining a healthy weight is a lifelong responsibility? As family members of someone with an intellectual disability (our son and brother, Jim), we offer this personal experience (with Jim's permission) as an example of trying different ways to get the message across while giving the responsibility, control, and informed choice-making skills to the person you support.

Jim had a significant weight problem when he was in his late teens and early twenties. Because he is just under 5 feet tall, if Jim gains only 1 extra pound it looks and feels more like 5. We worried that he would develop health problems related to his weight. For one, he often complained about sore hips. He didn't even seem to enjoy food so much as he felt compelled to consume it quickly. Jim has a moderate intellectual disability, so we believed we could talk to him about what he ate and how much, but the lure of fast food was impossible to fight. We are an active family, yet we found ourselves curtailing activities because Jim had difficulty going on hikes or other activities that required demanding physical exertion. This habit began to extend to others besides ourselves; we felt that if *we* had to hold back on our activities because of Jim's weight, it was pretty hard to ask students at the university where my husband Rick was a professor to include Jim in their weekend football pickup games, for instance. Our hearts would ache when we'd walk across campus on a Saturday afternoon while kids, some of them Rick's students, were out throwing the ball around. "That'd be fun," Jim would say. Even meeting a friend to take her dogs for an evening walk was sometimes too much exertion for Jim. We knew enough about "yo-yo" weight gain and loss that helping Jim lose and then maintain a healthy weight was going to mean sharing the decision-making with him.

Thus, *The Skinny Food, Fat Food Game* was born. Though no doubt some would argue against using value-laden words such as *skinny* and *fat*, we thought this was the most concrete way to provide Jim with basic information about food choice. The concept was pretty simple. I (Karin) drew a small illustration of Jim at the top of each of two pieces of 8½" × 11" bristol board. One showed him at a reasonable weight for his build. The other was an overweight Jim. In both drawings, he was smiling. We wanted to avoid the idea that he was bad or unhappy one way or the other. I laminated the bristol board. Then I set out to forage for food pictures in magazines, grocery store fliers, even the little recipe cards the grocery store offers as serving suggestions. Jim helped.

I cut out small photos of just about every food we came across: raw, cooked, canned, packaged, elegantly prepared, a full meal, condiment, sauce, you name it. I went beyond food and drink we regularly consumed at home because I knew that throughout his life, Jim would need to be able to make decisions about food in other people's homes, in restaurants, and other times he would be on his own. I cut out and pasted all of these pictures on construction paper backgrounds for better wear, separating the fat foods from the skinny foods by color (red=fat, green=skinny). Into a large red envelope that featured another drawing of Jim overweight, I instructed Jim to place the pictures of all of the high caloric, high fat foods that tend to cause a person to put on weight. Then he was to put pictures of all of the vegetables, fruits, fish, chicken, and lower caloric, lower fat items into a green envelope that showed Jim thin. I debated about creating another category so that something high calorie that was consumed in moderation could be considered an "in-between" food, but I thought that would complicate the message too much. Instead, the basic idea is that people can eat some foods and stay "skinny," whereas other foods will make people fat, and so they should be eaten in smaller portions.

Other, related rules were then easier to convey, such as some fat foods are only for special occasions (e.g., "We don't eat a whole birthday cake at one time or have birthday cake every day. Some foods are only for treats."). And a tricky little twist to learn is that you can have a perfectly good "skinny" food such as a baked potato, but you can turn it into a very "fat" food if you add butter, bacon bits, and sour cream. But salsa on a baked potato combines two "skinny" foods! Because there really isn't an ending, a game can last for 10 minutes or an hour.

Jim grasped the concepts related to this activity almost immediately. We called it a game so that the approach would be fun. Jim has taken the gaming aspect to heart and likes to trip up the other "player" by putting ALL of the "fat" food pictures on the "skinny" food page, arguing the validity of the placement with tongue firmly in cheek. But it was obvious he understood. We knew he was gaining some measure of control over decision making about food choices when he opted for a fruit selection at the salad bar instead of the soft ice cream machine. Now, when he talks about food he says things like "Cheesecake is good, but just a small one for a treat," and he's proud of his reputation as an excellent salad maker. "Salad is skinny food!" He takes the skin off his roast chicken so it becomes a skinny food. He looks for grocery items that are low fat or fat free. We occasionally go for a hamburger at a fast-food restaurant, and

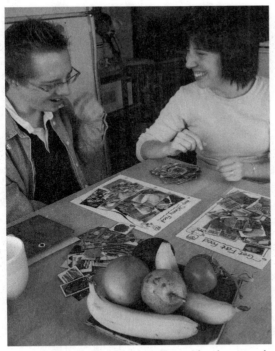

Friends Jim and Samantha have fun with a homemade game about healthy eating.

we've had to deal with a startled customer ahead of us when Jim pointed out, "Fat butt." We quickly explained to the customer that Jim was referring to the large fries and the consequences he would face if he ate too many, rather than to the customer's posterior.

Jim often asks if we'd like to play *Skinny Food, Fat Food*, and we are happy to comply. To keep it fresh, we continue to add new pictures. An unexpected side benefit of the game is that he can show other people how to play. His friend Samantha (pictured) says, "It's a great game. It's so much fun, and Jim has taught me a lot of things I didn't know. It's really interactive."

But the ultimate proof is in the pudding, as they say. Now weighing a steady 110 pounds, Jim lost at least 60 pounds since his peak weight in 1996. He's in control of his weight and eating habits. He runs with us. He can handle the exertion of his maintenance job at the YMCA. He enjoys picking out clothes that fit well, and he basks in compliments. He hasn't complained about sore hips in years. Obviously, all of this cannot be attributed to a little homemade game that helps him gain some measure of control over what he puts in his body, but it hasn't hurt. He can be as inclined as the rest of us to order battered fish and chips—and reminding him to eat more slowly is a constant—but he has a better chance of making good decisions most of the time. And it does our hearts good as he heads out the door with a weight-lifting buddy from the university and a football tucked under his arm.

Never use food as a reward. That doesn't mean one should never mark a special occasion with a celebration dinner or a chocolate shake. But to use food as a motivational tool to entice someone to do chores or behave in certain ways isn't a great idea. People are not pets. Similarly, denying food puts mealtime in the awkward position of punishment rather than enjoyable activity.

Supporting Choice Making

Shirley Gerein, director of a Canadian residential agency, says that for any of the staff who support people living in her agency, knowing how to support choice making is critical:

> *Even giving people some flexibility in when they eat is just a small way we can recognize the dignity of people. I like to ask if they would like to dish up their own food from the stove or if they'd like one of us to do it. If someone had a big lunch and doesn't feel like much supper, that's okay. If they'd like someone to come over for lunch, we help with the invitation. The little things like that is the difference between someone being treated with respect in their own home and the assumption that they are incapable.*

Gerein says many of the people in her agency lived for years, even decades, in institutions where they had few if any responsibilities around mealtime. Fortunately, this has changed in recent years as people have moved to more home-like community settings, and some of the residents enjoy helping out:

> *Mary is 65. She feels really good about helping out and if you compliment her, she always giggles. Everyone here enjoys having a choice of what to eat or what to have for dessert. Even something as small as doing your own dishes can be very satisfying.*

A little bit is infinitely more than nothing. Remember?

 Many kitchen appliances now come with independence-giving safety features, such as automatic shut-off kettles and coffee makers, cool-touch toasters, and bladeless electric can openers.

 Some microwaves come with pre-programmed buttons with pictures of the food along with the name to ensure appropriate cooking time. Stick the bag of popcorn in, close the door and hit the popcorn button.

AN ETHOS OF *"DOING FOR"* RATHER THAN *"DOING WITH"*

A fundamental shift in the attitudes of human service workers and agency policies in recent years has many people riding a teeter-totter of support for people with disabilities. Many agencies have embraced the idea that people with disabilities are growing, learning, changing human beings capable of looking after many of their own needs. This is a move away from the old medical model of care that perceived people with disabilities as passive recipients of service. Even though staff may understand the supported care approach, it's not always an easy change to put into practice.

Dr. Roger Stancliffe is a Senior Research Fellow with the Centre for Developmental Disability Studies, Royal Rehabilitation Centre, in Sydney, Australia. In a 2002 study that looked at 65 randomly selected people living in 34 group homes in New South Wales, Stancliffe, Dew, and Parmenter found an alarming lack of choice making and participation in domestic activities by people with disabilities:

> *In some residential services, there is conundrum for staff. They may not be recognized for involving residents with disabilities in everyday household chores and they may also be rebuked if domestic tasks are not completed satisfactorily. People with disabilities may not initiate and carry out activities on their own. Staff aren't supported to encourage their participation, so they accept nonparticipation and rationalize it as a choice on the part of the person with a disability.*
>
> *In Australia, there has also been a move away from providing staff with the teaching skills needed to support and teach residents to participate in these activities, including domestic and self-care activities, so there is very limited awareness among most staff about what it is possible for residents to [learn to] do. For example, low expectations combined with limited staff skills to alter the situation compounds the problem. There is definitely an ethos of doing for rather than doing with, and many staff see it as their job to care for residents rather than to assist them to participate and care for themselves with support. There are staff who perceive their jobs as being glorified domestics.*

In fact, Stancliffe has observed a tendency to focus on providing residents with "enjoyable activities in a sometimes shallow quest for quality of life but not necessarily real participation in everyday life."

Community outings (e.g., fast food, movies, bowling, vacations) with quite limited genuine social interaction are almost like the sugar-boost from a mid-afternoon candy bar. They provide some instant enjoyment, but left behind is a hollow hunger for something more substantial.

 Outside picnics are great if spilling is a concern. The birds and squirrels will thank you for it. Indoor "carpet picnics" are also great if sitting in a chair is challenging. Do it just for fun, and no need to worry about ants.

An Inspiring Model

The Centre for Developmental Disability Studies (CDDS) in Sydney is taking on the implementation and evaluation of a model developed in the United Kingdom called Active Support. Stancliffe is encouraged that the model has changed staff behavior and improved life for people with disabilities who live in group homes. Stancliffe explains,

> *One important feature of this model is that it gives significant attention to staff training and the procedural organization of a provision of support by staff. It is assumed that providing a normal environment is a necessary but not sufficient step for meaningful participation in activities. These activities must also involve well-organized support of individual residents, if satisfactory lifestyle outcomes are to be achieved. It seems clear that staff do not naturally do these things without training and support, and many agencies need to be provided with a coherent process and relevant training resources to bring this about effectively.*

Shirley Gerein describes it this way:

> *There are some Old Mother Hubbards in the residential system. They are wonderful people with great hearts who feel their job is to take care of people. As an agency, we have to actively train staff so that they become teachers and supporters, not do-fors.*

An Active Support model changes the role of the caregiver and their attitudes about themselves so that they are able to provide a higher proportion of assistance and praise for participation and greater engagement in activities. This new view also presents a very different image to the public of someone with a disability. According to Stancliffe:

> *Mealtime and all of the tasks related to it are such typical parts of everyday life that participation by people with disabilities contributes to their status as ordinary members of the community. Lining up at the supermarket checkout behind someone with a disability sends a powerful message to other shoppers that "this person is pretty much like me."*

 Asking for help in the corner market or grocery store is a good way to involve people in their local community. Remember to include everyone in the conversation so everyone interacts in whatever way they can.

I MADE IT MYSELF

Remember when you were given a bit of dough while one of your parents or grandparents rolled out a pie pastry? You fashioned it into shapes, sprinkled a pinch of sugar and some cinnamon on them, and while they baked, you peered through the window in the oven door, eagerly anticipating this masterpiece you had created. You were in total charge of those bits of pastry. You made them just the way you wanted. You *made* them. They were *yours*. Remember how that felt? Remember how they tasted?

People who once lived in institutions cite the ability to choose and have responsibilities around food as major accomplishments as they measure the benefits of a more independent life in the community. Ironically, the mundane routines of daily life that people without disabilities put up with, or at least take for granted, are the very milestones of independence raised when people with disabilities are asked what they enjoy most about their lives. Consider these personal stories:

I Wish Mom Coulda Seen Me Make a Cupcake

Darlene Leister spent 27 years in institutions. In 1988, the last institution she was in closed and she moved to a group home in a small prairie farming community. Seven years later, she moved into a supported apartment living program and enjoys her own place next to another unit where a friend with a disability lives.

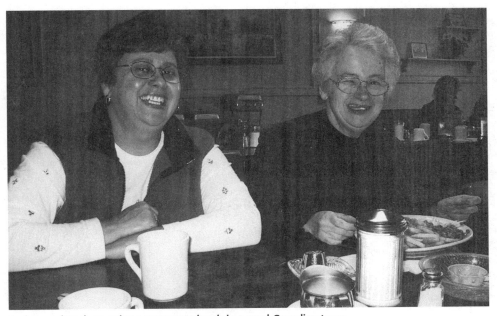

Audrey and Darlene enjoy a restaurant lunch in a rural Canadian town.

Oh, you bet, I enjoy it in my new home! I made Jell-O and I know how to do but-ter tarts. We made cupcakes once, and I put a cherry on top and we iced 'em. And I never done that in North Park Centre! I was so happy I got to load the dish-washer. That was so thrilling, and I never done that before neither. I learned how to can cherries and beet pickles, cucumbers, crab apples, and jam . . . Somebody gave us all the crab apples and beets and that. We did relish, too, we ground stuff up and turned the thing and made relish. I never done it before. (as cited in Melberg Schwier, 1990, pp. 99, 103)

Darlene later told us, "I wish my Mom and Dad coulda seen me make a cupcake. They passed away, you know. But they woulda been real proud."

Pass the Pasta, Per Favore

Andrea was eating this horrible homogenized stuff every day, just brown, all the same texture—and then it started. One day he just went to one of his mates and asked if he could try some of his food. Then he just tried something else, then something else. He is still not a big eater but this progress is very good. And when he decided to start eating, it is changing so much from one day to the next. All of a sudden he would like to have some pizza, a crusty pizza and that's all he wanted and then pasta and that was a happy day. I thought maybe it was a dream. —Edi Cecchini, Italy

Just Equals

I always enjoy seeing Laura take charge of her decisions. She orders her own meal and interacts with the waiter or waitress. I think her decision-making is a bit limited in the group home, so when we're out in the world, it's good for her to have some con-trol. I'm always learning something from Laura as I observe the way she manages in the world. Something I've really noticed is that there are times when she's been frus-trated and upset in situations where she's the one being told what to do or what she can't do. When she gets frustrated, it's like she's a teenager who gets angry when they feel grown up but can't make their own decisions. But with me, I'm not a group home staff or anyone who is there to correct her or teach her. We're just friends, equals. I've really found out how rich and interesting she is as a person. If she wants to make certain food choices when we're together, that's her choice. I'm not staff and I think when we get together for mealtime, it's sort of a freedom for her. —Rory Hoover, United States

Murrandah Steers the Menu

I, for example, don't get punkin, which is my favorite. Murrandah won't eat punkin. He'll just spit it out so the wife, she don't cook it so I don't get punkin. So we eat a lot of pasta because Murrandah enjoys pasta. Rice. Potatoes he likes. He won't drink milk. When he was a baby, he had the tube, you know. A lot of things over the years we just cut out of what we eat. And we all cook, even me and the young fella Paul, and when we cook we just have in mind what Murrandah likes. And with five kids in the house, it's just not worth it. The other kids end up getting all upset because Murrandah gets to have custard rice and they have to have steak, if you can believe that. So we mainly just eat what we have in mind for him. He really enjoys the Wiggles, those blokes on TV that jump around and sing for kids. We buy cans of baked beans and that with the Wiggles on it. We show him the label and then he'll eat it. So it's up to him, I reckon. —Goomblar Wylo, Australia

There's More to Meals than Cooking

We're not really the cooking sort. We don't cook. At all, really. I think we'd both rather have a relaxing dinner and let someone else do the cooking. Our conversations are very fluid at mealtime. I'm always impressed with the way Laura handles things and I always learn something from her. Laura really likes sports. In fact, we went to a stadium for a hockey game, and I didn't know she was afraid of heights. We were loaded down with our hot dogs and drinks, and I was trying to help her get up in the stands and it occurred to me she was afraid to go up into the bleachers. But she was determined to overcome that and get up there to see the game. She really helps me understand what she has to go through to be in the world. I manage a volunteer program, but that's a different interaction than being a friend. —Rory Hoover, United States

Good Things Come to Those Who Wait

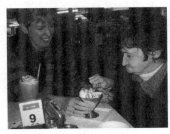

Australian sisters Beth (left) and Margie share some ice cream during an afternoon visit.

We've been exploring what Margie likes eating. We did try offering her fish and chips, but she turned down the chips. I make a good homemade muesli and I offered that to her for breakfast, not really thinking she'd like it. But she did enjoy it. It's a matter of trial and error. We sometimes offer her a choice of breakfast cereals; we line them up and ask her, 'Which one would you like?' I've been watching Doris, a wonderful staff person where Margie lives, who gives Margie a choice and then is willing to wait. She says, 'Do you want this one or that one?' Margie often says yes to both and Doris just waits. Finally Margie reaches for one. Doris just allows more time, whereas I tend to give up and think well, she doesn't understand what I'm asking her so I'll decide for her. That's something that I still have to learn. —Beth Macleod, Australia

Do you have snacks available in the cupboard or refrigerator that people can help themselves to if they feel the munchies coming on? This is an adult privilege most of us take for granted, but something that may be denied to an adult with a disability.

We Do It Our Own Selves

Mostly I clean up my messes before and after we eat when I get it on the table for me and Myrna. My parents taught me to clean up the kitchen and you won't get germs. I don't wanna be sick. I been healthy for the last 25 years, and we wanna keep it that way. There are all different sizes of grocery and we look at prices before we buy them. We pick the lowest price because of my budget and my wife's budget. We don't follow what other people make their rules and we make our own rules and when we hungry and when we not hungry. My wife and I can't afford to buy fancy meals. All we can afford to buy in our budget, certain food for myself and my wife Myrna. —James Necula, Canada

Thinking It Through

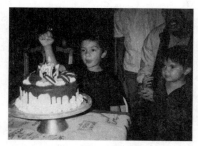

The Chou brothers admire Michael's birthday cake; Uncle Anthonike reminds Daniel he can look but not eat. He'll have his own version of his brother's birthday treat.

Danny likes very plain food. McDonald's french fries are a favorite. The texture is very even and feels the same. He is very particular about touch. If he falls down in the yard, he uses the back of his hands to push himself up. The feel of McDonald's fries is acceptable to him. He's still too young to really understand that there are some things he can't have. I have a friend whose son can't have eggs. Instead of just telling him no, if he says, 'Oh, can I have some cake?' she will say, "Yes, that looks good. But do you think it has eggs in it?' And her son will think and decide there are eggs, so he can't have that. She's letting him work out what he can and can't have. —Leigh Chou, United States

Recognizing the Need for Some Control

There are lots of very subtle barriers for Kahurangi. All of them look like bad manners. He doesn't like to share at a kai* table. He likes his space. At the moment, there are developmental reasons; he's growing, he's gangly. But he's never liked being crowded unless he's the one doing the crowding. He does cheerfully accept cuddles from his immediate whanau,** but he prefers to be the one giving them, the one in control. Sitting at a crowded table is very stressful. Sometimes he'll leave, but if I bully him into being there, he will wear one of his faces, particularly the one where his eyebrows crawl down to the end of his nose. Very attractive. He can't stand the clatter of knives on forks and I don't blame him. He also can't stand being told when to be hungry. His father, George, does the main food preparation these days since he's the

*food
**family

one doing the home schooling. He's found it easier to prepare the main meal of the day at lunchtime, which consists of, at the moment, broccoli for the younger child and either beans, corn on the cob, or potatoes for Kahurangi. That's what he wants . . . He's been a happy and serene child for over a year now, so why risk changing it. —Bronwyn Thurlow, New Zealand

 Always be respectful of personal space.

And This One's Just Right

Danny's a really picky food eater. He's got some particular foods he likes. He misses cheese, but he'd be very happy with white rice, peanut butter, and jelly for every meal. For a while, he was very resistant to odd textures, especially in food. It had to feel right. Pudding or anything like it was out. Rice was good. He'd eat with his hands. The spoon had a feel to it at first, but now he uses it. He'd just look at food and push the plate away or turn away from it. We didn't pressure him; we'd try to give him what he would tolerate. —Leigh Chou, United States

 For someone who has difficulty scooping, try a swivel spoon. These spoons have a swivel mechanism that helps individuals without much control in their wrists to eat their own meals without dumping food.

I Got Ideas

I got a million of cooking ideas in my head. I could be one of those cooking guys on TV, but they probably wouldn't pay me any money. I try not to make anything real fancy so I can lose a little more weight. When I make a fancy meal, her mother give me heck on why you feed my daughter so much she get fat! I think Myrna is real pretty. I say I get started in the kitchen and I can't stop! I get all the ideas from a restaurant where I used to work at. —James Necula, Canada

They're Just Biscuits

Finally, here's a story from Karin's own experience.

One winter afternoon, my 29-year-old son Jim asked if we could make baking powder biscuits. I was pleased with his initiative and we pulled out the easy recipe (see p. 204) and assembled the ingredients. Jim donned his apron. Within 15 minutes, I'm embarrassed to say, I morphed into the *Seinfeld* Soup Nazi. My only saving grace is that I fell just short of grabbing the bowl away from him, shrieking, "Oh, it'll be easier if I just do it myself!" He wasn't measuring right. He wasn't mixing right. He was messy. He was adding ingredients out of order. He made the biscuits too big, then too small. They were too close together on the baking sheet. For goodness sake, they're only biscuits; what's the worst that could happen? Well, the worst did happen. What could have been a lovely hour or so spent together in the warmth of our kitchen was ruined because I was more concerned—no, entirely consumed—by some bizarre self-imposed sense of quality control rather than being with my son. I apologized and the next day, we tried again. He put on his favorite Beatles CD, read the recipe card, and decided to add raisins and orange zest to make a biscuit/scone hybrid. We got flour on the floor and ended up with the most un-uniform globs of dough to ever enter the oven. With a cup of tea, a little strawberry jam, a helping of crow for me, and my son's huge self-satisfied and forgiving grin, they were perfect.

Food. Making it yourself can be a hallmark of adulthood.—Karin Melberg Schwier, Canada

---

 Make a conscious effort to leave your "teacher" self behind from time to time. Let things go. Let there be times when you just enjoy each other. We call them "No Nag Days."

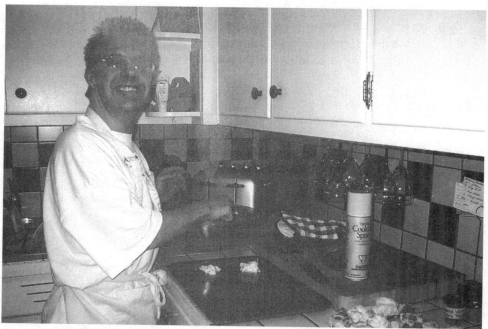

Jim makes biscuits. They may not be perfect, but they are his!

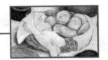

CHAPTER 7

The Experience
of Disability
and Dining

GARY McPHERSON

Up until October 2, 1955, my eating experiences were like any other normal, active, 9-year-old boy. Then, I contracted poliomyelitis. Polio.

From that day on, my experiences with eating and dining were significantly influenced by my altered physical condition. Polio left me respirator-ventilator dependent with quadriplegia. This means that I am dependent on a ventilator for breathing assistance, particularly at night, and that all four of my limbs have varying degrees of paralysis. Over the years, I've learned a voluntary method of breathing called glossopharyngeal breathing, which allows me to function independently away from the respirator for several hours a day. Why is this important in relation to dining? I consciously have to breathe, and it makes it somewhat more difficult to chew and swallow at the same time. Sometimes, this extra effort can affect the quality of my eating experience.

I'm sure all of us experience changes in our dining experiences as we age and as our circumstances in life change. I'm no different. For the first 9 years of my life, I grew up in a relatively normal family environment before becoming a resident of the University of Alberta hospital. In 1974, I moved to the Aberhart Centre [then a long-term, University-affiliated medical care center in Edmonton, Alberta] before getting married and moving out into the community in 1989. The experiences that I'm about to share were significantly influenced by my residential environment, my roommates, staff, friends, volunteers, and family. It has been an interesting inward journey as I search for the words to describe the various eating and dining experiences that have contributed so richly to my life.

After contracting polio, eating was somewhat uncomfortable in the sense that breathing and eating in an iron lung were not always compatible. One of the main reasons was that the swallowing sometimes provided a slight irritation that exacerbated my ongoing breathing difficulties. I know that at one time I used to say, "I eat to live,

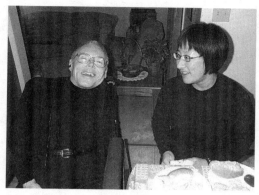

Gary enjoys mealtime with his wife, Valerie.

not live to eat." Fortunately, things progressed and eating became more than just putting food into my mouth to sustain life.

When I transferred from the Royal Alexandra Hospital to Station 32 in the University Hospital on October 15, 1955, it not only changed my living environment but also the quality of my eating experiences. Over time, as the population on the polio ward changed, my interactions with my newfound roommates and colleagues began to provide me with more enjoyment through eating. Mealtimes became an opportunity to interact, share stories, swap lies, and generally interject humor into what at times was a personally challenging existence. However, if it were not for the quality of the human exchange, mealtimes would not be very memorable because the food was often unrecognizable. My mother was an excellent cook, and at times I think this made it more difficult for me to adjust to the overcooked vegetables, leather-like roast beef, and inferior-quality instant potatoes served on the ward.

One particular moment that I remember clearly occurred just a few days after my interhospital transfer. I was lying in my iron lung and trying to make myself understood about something or other. Because of my particular condition at the time, I did not have use of my voice and people needed to read my lips in order to understand my particular needs. I was trying to communicate a message, and whoever was reading my lips was not quite getting it. That person kept asking me if I was asking for "T-bone steak?" Getting somewhat frustrated, I kept trying to communicate something other than that, but the person kept saying, "T-bone steak." After the third time, I suddenly got smart and said, "Yes!" Within hours, my mother and father arrived with a freshly cooked and tasty T-bone steak. I don't remember what I originally wanted, but I do remember that the T-bone steak was better than what I was asking for at the time.

In the fall of 1957 the polio ward was moved to Station 67, a brand-new area within the University Hospital. I lived in a large room with as many as seven other resident patients, and we all needed to be fed because most of us did not have the ability to physically feed ourselves. The meal experience was sometimes complicated by a lack of staff; this meant that one person would feed at least two people and as many as four at one time.

It all began with the food wagon arriving at a set time. From there, the various food trays were sorted by room and individual and transferred to a stretcher with wheels. At least one staff member who was assigned to a particular room would push the stretcher and wheel the meals to the appropriate area. This was the pre-preparation that went into virtually every cold or lukewarm meal that I had while living in the University Hospital. Thinking back on it, there were some foods there I enjoyed:

bacon (when it was crisp), pork chops, certain soups, hot dogs, hamburgers, french fries, and desserts. You can see that I used to eat a fairly unhealthy diet. I'm pleased to say that my eating choices of today are almost the polar opposite.

But despite the usually bad food, this is where memorable moments started, and it began with warm interactions between roommates, staff, and whoever was involved in that particular meal. Jokes were told, daily experiences were shared, social plans were made, business ideas were hatched, and the seeds of future dreams were planted. It was also a time to console someone who had experienced a personal loss, as was needed from time to time. For the most part, I remember these mealtimes as times of warmth and friendliness.

In September 1974, those of us who remained in the University Hospital moved to the Aberhart Centre, a smaller satellite facility that was operated by the University Hospital administration. Initially, it was built as a treatment facility for those individuals who had contracted tuberculosis (TB). By the time we moved to the Aberhart, TB had been brought under control with treatment and medications. This meant that the population of the former sanatorium had now changed from what was its primary focus.

The entire eating experience at the Aberhart was influenced by the fact that, historically speaking, patients with TB were provided with a high-quality diet. Even considering that the internal population of the Aberhart had fewer patients with TB now that we had moved, the quality of food was noticeably better than the quality of the University hospital food. In part, this was due to the fact that it was easier to cook smaller quantities, as well as keep it warm until it was actually consumed. Moving to the Aberhart was akin to moving to a small town from a large city, and it also meant that everybody knew everybody. This seemed to have a beneficial effect on the overall eating experience within the Aberhart. It even helped make vegetables taste like vegetables!

In contrast to the large wards/rooms that we lived in at the University, the Aberhart living facility provided each resident with more privacy. Most often there were two of us in one room, and on occasion there was only one in a room. This privacy had a considerable impact on the Aberhart dining experience: We no longer ate together. Generally speaking, Aberhart was a very good environment to live in when compared with the University Hospital. But even though the food was better, the actual Aberhart dining experience lacked the camaraderie and warmth that was so apparent previously. Accordingly, the spin-off benefits of mealtime interaction were lessened through the Aberhart migration. The human interaction was usually limited to staff to resident dialogue, and was influenced by the level of rapport between the one who was being fed and the staff member who was doing the feeding.

Soon after getting polio, it seemed important to regain as much physical independence as possible. This was a time of intensive physiotherapy and experimentation. My quest to be as independent as I could be yielded some hard-learned lessons. For example, I was fitted with an elaborate sling that was attached to my wheelchair. The sling supported my left arm and hand so that I could physically feed myself from a tray top that was attached to my chair. I soon realized that the required energy to feed myself combined with my breathing difficulties created more problems than solutions. I made a decision to use my limited energy in a much more focused way. I had grown beyond the need to prove my physical independence and manhood through the act of feeding myself to the point of exhaustion.

As I grew into my teens, I was somewhat self-conscious about how I looked. This in turn affected me when I went out into the public, and often I wouldn't eat. Simply not eating out was a way to avoid drawing attention to the fact that I needed to be physically fed by someone else. Besides that, eating and breathing for me were still a chore. To some degree, this self-consciousness carried over into my early years of dating, when I was lucky enough to get one! Dating was often complicated by the need to coordinate transportation and access. Fortunately, I had friends to help me out with the occasional ride when necessary, but often the desired place for a meal was not accessible to a wheelchair user. Also, I needed to get over the fact that my date for the evening would have to feed me, or she would be eating alone. Eventually, I learned to turn that dependency to my advantage. It became an opportunity to enjoy each other's company and the conversation that comes with it.

Something that happened on a regular basis when dining out, and it still does, is the interaction (or lack of it) that I have with the server on initial contact. The waiter or waitress quickly reveals their personal level of comfort in dealing with me as a person who has an obvious disability. It is not uncommon for the person that I am with to be asked, "What does he want to eat?" At that point, I usually respond. Years ago, this lack of acknowledgment of me as a person bothered me, but I've since learned that it is my responsibility to make people as comfortable with me as I can. Unfortunately, not all people who are in my position handle the situation with sensitivity. Like it or not, I am an ambassador for the person who comes after me. The impression I leave will make a difference for others. I have experienced the reverse because someone with a disabling condition or his or her companion responded to a situation with anger or sarcasm. When I came along, it was assumed I'd act the same way.

As a dining patron, physical access to the building is one of my primary considerations, although I will occasionally dine at a location where steps are involved. Increasingly, as the population ages and more wheelchairs become visible, businesses and restaurants are demonstrating sensitivity to the needs of a variety of patrons, me included. Over the years, in order to access a variety of eating establishments, including some of the best, I have often had to go through a circuitous route in order to get to the main dining area. Consequently, I have seen many back halls and the inside of kitchen facilities en route. Occasionally, this has given me an added benefit to understanding the preparation that goes into making a meal. Other than that, my experience probably mirrors that of most dining patrons.

Eating, mealtimes, and dining have provided me with some of my most memorable moments. These moments were gathered amidst a varied environment, and were always fueled by the conversation and warmth of human interaction. Most of my eating experiences have been positive. However, I have always been affected by smoking and secondhand smoke. I'm sure that my breathing difficulties don't make it any more palatable to me. During my hospital stay, when a staff member had residual smoking effects like stained fingers or smelled of cigarettes, it affected the quality of my eating experience and still does today.

I have certainly developed a sense of humor over the years to help deal with a variety of mealtime experiences, both positive and negative. I recall the time when my son Jamie was 3 years old and my wife Valerie was preparing a meal of spaghetti and tomato sauce. I don't know whether you have ever tried to reason with a 3-year-old, but usually I had little success. On this occasion, Jamie insisted that he wanted to feed his dad. I said to Valerie, "I need the largest tea towel that you have, please!" Jamie climbed up onto my lap and proceeded to feed me. He did a pretty good job for the most part, but I'm sure that if I had had tonsils they would've been removed during one or two particularly enthusiastic forkfuls.

Over the years, in addition to Jamie, I have had hundreds of different people feed me a variety of meals. One of the things that I've noticed is that people have a tendency to reflect their personal eating preferences in the way that they feed me. For example, some people like to eat their vegetables first and others like to eat them last. Some people like to eat slowly; others like to eat fast. Often at mealtimes, the person who is feeding me also eats at the same time. In my brother's case, I can tell when he is hungry because the food comes slowly. Only after he has had several bites does it come my way more frequently. Until he gets food in his own tummy, he seems almost oblivious to the fact that I might be hungry as well. In contrast, I can tell when my wife is hungry because the food comes fast and furiously. I need to suggest that she slow down so that I can breathe.

Finally, though I am a father and husband, I have yet to actually cook a meal. However, it has occurred to me to study the culinary arts and attempt to address this domestic shortcoming through the physical cooperation of a willing son or daughter. Like many things in my life, this is on my "to do" list.

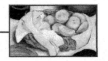

CHAPTER 8

Mallory and the Circle Girls

Good Food, Good Friends, Good Gossip

BARB HORNER

Like most teenagers, Mallory Horner loves to eat. Her favorite place to be is in the thick of things in the kitchen, gossiping with a circle of girlfriends her age, listening to the sounds of food preparation and smelling the aroma of great culinary delights.

When Mallory was in fourth grade, her father and I initiated a circle of friends for her and planned monthly get-togethers at our home. Over the years, Mallory's Circle has evolved, with some friends moving on to other interests and new friends becoming involved. Some of Mallory's friends have known her since primary school and others since junior high [middle school] and now high school. The Circle Girls meet every 2 weeks at the Horner house and are involved in the planning process and menu now more than ever. But what's more fun for the girls than just meeting at Mallory's is being away from home with their friends, where they can cook and eat what they like.

During the past three summers, Mallory heads off with the Circle Girls and her personal support worker to vacation away from family. While at camp, Mallory and her friends make good use of the large kitchen and especially enjoy the walk-in fridge where they go to cool down when the weather is hot. At camp, they realize that identifying daily menus, preparing food, and eating meals together brings them closer as a group. Even though Mallory has many challenges, her friends realize how important Mallory's diet is and how much she truly loves to eat—about as much as they do!

When they gather to make something to eat, the girls talk about many things such as whether the meals are healthy, and they try to balance junk food and sweets with the good stuff. They enjoy taste testing what they are cooking, and Jesse ponders, "How much can I eat during preparation?" They all wonder how and when they can fit chocolate into their day. The girls realize how important it is to develop teamwork in the kitchen so everyone has a task and is involved. Karen says, "When everyone's together, we socialize and share ideas and vent when necessary." Becky pipes up, "Everybody talks, and when we do all of our voices get louder. Mallory often laughs

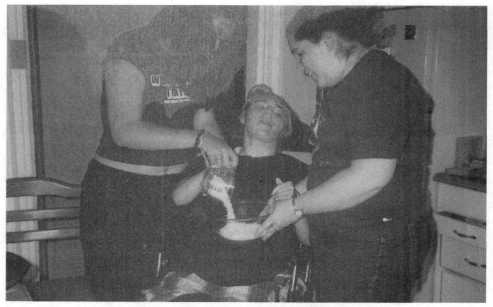

Becky, Mallory, and Jesse get into the stirring action on a batch of pancakes.

at us. I think she gets so excited with all of our chatter. Mallory is involved and likes to be in the kitchen to listen to all of the sounds and smell all of the mouth-watering smells." . . . "When we're all in the kitchen together," Jesse adds, "it's relaxing even though it's work." No one gets left out. That's a life lesson the girls have taken from the kitchen into the rest of their lives.

Mallory is generally in the thick of things. She loves the kitchen and participates by often just being present and by being vocal. Mallory relies mainly on her auditory senses and loves the clatter of dishes, running water, the sound of the microwave, and the inevitable conversation that happens naturally when a group of young women are in the kitchen together. She expresses herself vocally and adds her two cents' worth. She can hold bowls on her lap and spoons in her hands, and with assistance she can stir things or use her switch to operate the blender or food processor. She can help set the table and assist with drying the dishes. She excels as the number one food taster, probably her favorite job.

Mallory's friends and personal support worker assist her to eat, and when they are away together it seems that whomever is closest to Mallory at the time generally is the one to offer her her meal. The Circle Girls enjoy their get-togethers in the summer, and throughout the year they come to the Horner house every couple of weeks to hang out. The girls identify some of their favorite foods they like to share together. Mallory has a sweet tooth and appreciates anything to do with chocolate—her facial expression and soft cooing of gratitude clearly show how much she enjoys such treats. Karen appreciates "lots of junk food, pickles, and pizza with lots of meat"; Jesse likes Mallory's mom's homemade chocolate cake, chili, hot dogs, and burgers; Gwen just enjoys pretzels; Becky loves homemade lasagna, chips, and salsa; Susan likes Taco Night. They all agree that "it all tastes so good and it tastes better because we're all together having a great time."

Becky says, "We enjoy getting together because we are all in different classes and grades and when we come to Mallory's, sometimes we haven't talked or seen each other for awhile. We have lots to catch up on and lots to say." They appreciate coming to Mallory's home so that they have this important time together as a group. They are extremely social creatures; they love to gab. They might gossip a bit and the more they talk, the louder their voices get. Mallory so enjoys all of this interaction and is in her glory when she shares good food and good gossip with her good friends. Mallory's expresses her delight at these times with her body language and her gleeful vocalization.

For future get-togethers at Mallory's house, the girls think they would like to have some theme nights for diverse cultural experiences that would include food, props and decorations, costumes (maybe), and music (definitely). Then everyone really gets to enjoy the full experience in every way. Mallory relies on her other senses to truly enjoy and appreciate such experiences, so having music to listen to, food to taste, and costumes to wear and feel assists Mallory to fully enjoy the moment. Karen suggests a Hawaiian Night with beach clothes, Hawaiian pizza, and umbrella drinks. Susan thinks they should plan an evening to enjoy Asian food with music and perhaps a movie. Most of the girls think it's time for another overnight pajama party—but that's more fun when Mallory's parents are away, so timing is everything. The group is looking ahead to a Halloween Party with Mallory; their theme as a group is Christmas. They will be tree ornaments, decorations, and gifts, and Mallory will be the tree.

There is nothing like the combination of food, teenagers, and music, and Mallory thrives when in the company of her friends. As her parents, we only have to look at her face to see that she loves being part of the Circle Girls—at least as much as she enjoys chocolate. And that's a lot.

AN INTIMATE A-FARE

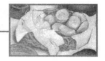

CHAPTER 9

Comfort Food, Comfort Context

Food, like a loving touch
or a glimpse of divine power,
has that ability to comfort.
—NORMAN KOLPAS

From morning till night, sounds drift from the kitchen,
most of them familiar and comforting. . . . On days when
warmth is the most important need of the human heart, the kitchen is
the place you can find it, it dries the wet sock, it cools the hot little brain . . .
—E.B. WHITE (AS CITED IN CRONKHITE, 2003)

When we ask our son/brother Jim to list his favorite foods, it's clear that the context surrounding those foods is as important as the food itself. He recites a list and every food item is associated with family, friends, and occasions:

Chicken breast, 'nember? And turkey. At Thanksgiving Maddy and Grandpa's.
And mash potato. Pumpkin pie. Dressing. Tomato soup. For lunch, I make it,
and cheese sandwich I do by myself. [Vietnamese] roll things. At Norm's for
Fringe [Festival] on the street. Bagel. From Superstore, I pick it out. My job.
House white. On Friday, we walk to have glass of wine. Popcorn and some
grapefruit. For movies, rent it from Blockbuster. Steak. I barbeque with Rick my
dad, back deck for summertime. Fish chips. Australia and New Zealand, my
29 birthday Christchurch. Momo cookies Christmas [sent by his grandmother
"Momo" and grandfather "Bobo" from Florida]. Biscuits. I make it myself, my
apron on, CD music on. Salad. My job, I do good job, small pieces for tomato,
zucchini, and green pepper. Just small. I'm good at that, 'nember? That's it.

Comfort food is not necessarily comforting without the context. What happens around a meal and with whom is just as important, sometimes maybe more so. Nicola Schaefer, whose daughter Catherine requires total assistance, says her daughter was never far from the kitchen as she was growing up:

> I'd be at the sink, chopping up this and that for supper and I'd make sure she'd be there, in her chair, beside me. Sometimes it was just to keep her from being run over by her rambunctious brothers. We'd have a lovely chat. I'd put a few bits on her tray so she could feel them. She couldn't help in the sense of chopping things up for me, but she could moosh them around on her tray. She could smell all the lovely smells in the kitchen as things were cooking and I'd talk about the day. The point was, really, that she was there. I know she quite enjoyed that, the being there.

 Learn what kinds of foods make people happy. Is there a special birthday cake that brings back wonderful childhood memories?

Adam is a young man with significant cerebral palsy. He lived in a residential home in San Diego, California, where the operators, Dorrie and Richard, were like parents to the children. Then-college student Erin (one of the authors) volunteered to be a surrogate sister. She recalls that while the food was classic down-home cooking, there were contexts in the fast-food realm that couldn't be beat:

> Adam loved french fries. But really, I think Adam loved what french fries meant to him even more. Rarely did Dorrie ever make french fries at home, but once a week after Adam had therapy, Richard would take him to McDonald's for some. He would get to go see his therapists, whom he loved, and then afterward he and Richard would always go for a "secret" trip for french fries together. It was an occasion for them to spend a couple of quality hours together. The joke between them was that it had to be a "secret" because he may spoil his dinner. Adam would always come home with a huge mischievous grin, smelling like a french fry himself. He would wait for me to ask the inevitable. "Did you have french fries again?" or "Does someone smell like a french fry in here?" That was always his cue and he would start laughing so hard, he'd go into extensor posturing and almost pop right out of his wheelchair. The ritual over for another week, we'd all sit down to dinner (which was never spoiled!) and continue with the evening's routine.

Social isolation is probably one of the most debilitating barriers for people with disabilities, particularly for those who rely on others—staff, family, volunteers, or friends—to keep them connected to community. Research has indicated that there exists a relatively high percentage of adults with disabilities "who never visit family or friends outside their own residence in a given month, do not engage in social activities inside their own residence . . . in a given week, do not converse by telephone in a given week" (L'Institut Roeher Institute, 1995, p. 206). Many more cope with periodic isolation. To be more precise, says Cam Crawford, President, L'Institut Roeher Institute in Toronto, data from the 1991 Health and Activity Limitation Survey (HALS) show that the total number of people age 15 years and older with disabilities was 3,533,000. Of these, 315,000 adults with disabilities (9% of all adults with disabilities) never attend social activities or visit with family or friends. Of these, 147,000 people (4% of all adults with disabilities) will never attend or take part in community activities such as religious and related activities, volunteer work, going to sporting events, concerts, plays, movies, museums, libraries, art galleries, parks, or seminars. Approximately 40,000 of these people (1.1% of all adults with disabilities) will never talk with others by telephone, and 20,000 of these people (0.6% of all adults with disabilities) consider themselves housebound (i.e., restricted to their personal home). Data from the previous 1986 HALS tell much the same story (C. Crawford, personal communication, 2004).

June Isaacson Kailes is a disability policy consultant and the Associate Director, Center for Disability Issues and the Health Professions, Western University of Health Sciences in Pomona, California. She believes that these statistics haven't improved much largely because it is still assumed that the needs of people with disabilities are somehow "special" and different from those of others:

> *Including people with disabilities in all aspects of life isn't just a "special interest" issue. Accommodating people with disabilities often translates into being better equipped to serve all people. People with disabilities are no more "special" in our need for contact with others and access to community than anyone else. There are, however, more environmental, physical, and communication barriers that can limit our ability to connect.*

 The Golden Rule of "Do unto others as you would have them do unto you" applies to your dining experiences.

Some agencies that support people with disabilities are paying attention to the need for people in their services to connect to community. Some are encouraging more deliberate reflection on current levels of social inclusion experienced by residents. In Nova Scotia, Canada, a tool called Essential Connections is used by the Regional Residential Services Society to help staff consider questions concerns as these:

Whether a resident has quality peer relationships (non-paid and non-volunteer), whether he or she periodically invites a friend or romantic partner over for dinner, and/or whether he or she engages in recreational activities with peers on the weekend. The answers to such questions are likely to reveal that even among those who are not totally "socially isolated," the majority experience low levels of social inclusion. (Regional Residential Services Society, 1998, p. 39).

Whitaker (1989) suggested that, for people with profound disabilities, several elements can determine a high quality of life. They include

- Useful skills (e.g., holding a cup)
- A variety of stimulating experiences in a comfortable environment
- Opportunities to exercise choice
- Caring relationships

We think it's so important for caregivers and anyone who is spending mealtimes with people who have disabilities to see it as not just a time to "get the person fed" or a chore, but a warm time of interaction. Children (and adults) who take their meals through a tube still can have mealtimes that are rich in communication and contact. "Your touch, voice, and care will help your child associate a positive feeling with [mealtime] rather than regarding it as just another procedure that happens frequently throughout the day" (Medlen, 2002, p. 39).

A quality mealtime enhances a person's quality of life. Food, good company, and an attentive mealtime really do have healing powers if given the chance.

 Come to the kitchen or the table ready to be emotionally devoted to being with that person for this time. Your mealtime companion deserves your total attention.

WHAT'S FOR DINNER?

As friends and caregivers, do we ever ask family members what may be the person's favorite, something that may be longed for, but out of reach? How often are people with disabilities asked about their own vestiges of childhood comfort, or discomfort for that matter? How often do we say, "Is there something you'd really like to have for dinner this weekend?" Are residential staff bound by agency policy on bulk grocery purchases or do they ever turn to someone with a disability served by the agency to ask, "Have you ever thought about some new food you'd really like to try? Did your mom or dad ever cook anything that you really loved and haven't had for years? Just name it, and we'll make it together."

People sometimes describe their favorite foods in terms of what they would request for their "last meal." To Robert Perske, this is not just a hypothetical idea. Perske has been tirelessly supporting people with intellectual disabilities on death row in the United States—people he's convinced were coerced into giving false confessions. He recalls mealtime for Joe Arridy in Canon City, Colorado. Warden Best saw that Joe got ice cream for his last three meals. Joe was overjoyed at this opportunity because he didn't really understand death (Perske, 1995). At the time this book was published, another man, Richard Lapointe, was also pinning his hopes on Perske and a few others who believed he did not commit murder and were working to get him freed. Richard had a daydream that kept him going: "He's looking forward to what he's going to have when we win the appeal and he gets out of prison," says Perske. He adds:

> We talk about it a lot, sort of like we GIs used to discuss food over and over again in the Philippines during WWII. A couple of others and I are taking Richard for lobster. One of the finest seafood places in the Boston Harbor area is only about a mile away from MacDougall Correctional Institution. We talk about how we're going to meet him at the front gate when it's all over and we'll walk the mile to that restaurant. Last time I saw him, Richard explained for a good 15 minutes to this Colorado-Kansas-Nebraska midlander all the techniques one must use in order to enjoy a lobster dinner. Afterward, we'll watch his favorite Red Sox play at Fenway Park. It's going to be a pilgrimage to his First Meal. Not the last meal on death row, but the first meal when he's free. It's a colorful, wonderful dream that keeps us all looking forward.

So, what do you want to do for dinner?
How often do we ask?

No One Recipe

No hard-and-fast rules dictate what a mealtime experience should be for every person with a disability. Don't make assumptions about someone based on disability, diagnosis, or even first impression. Everyone and every circumstance is different. What is essential, however, is to break bread with someone as an equal.

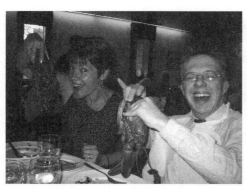

Trying new foods is always fun, even when it looks like it might bite back.

Half of the success in throwing a great dinner party comes from matching people who will enjoy each other's company, so find out what makes people tick. We don't mean a checklist; mealtimes are much more dynamic and organic. Most people with disabilities don't require any help out of the ordinary. Just because someone has cerebral palsy, it doesn't mean a mealtime companion will have to do A, B, and C to ensure an enjoyable experience. True, some disabilities pose particular challenges, but don't assume all people with cerebral palsy, for example, require the same thing at mealtime.

Once we start looking at the variety of activities and tasks involved in mealtime, including preparing for it, consuming it, and its aftermath, it's easier to involve someone with a disability in many different ways. Even ordering a pizza involves an array of decision-making skills, communications, abilities, and preferences, and the adventure of trying new things.

 Try playing some nice music while you're cooking and eating.

 If you decide to light a candle for more atmosphere at the dining table, remember that candles with strong odors may not only interfere with the taste pleasures but also may cause respiratory problems, so get nonscented candles.

It is vital to remember to keep going back to the most important thing. We call it "checking the pantry." Whether you are just getting to know someone or are interested in knowing the person better, get to know who, what, when, why, and how. Review who this person is (as a human being, not as a diagnosis). Talk to people close to the person. Does she have favorite memories from childhood with food and circumstances you can help recreate? Are there practical things you will need to know in order to be with this person in a relaxed way that allows for comfortable interaction? Remember, you're entering into or participating in this not as a job, but as a chance for a connection.

TIPS FOR BECOMING A BETTER MEALTIME PARTNER

Keep the following questions in mind when you are preparing to spend time with someone who has a disability. Each person is unique, so don't feel the following constitutes a set of "rules" or a checklist necessary for everyone:

- Who are you dining with?
- What sorts of things does the person like?
- What do you have in common?
- What are some things to talk about?
- When will you be meeting? Is it for a quick lunch? A longer dinner?

- Do you need to worry about a schedule? Is there an activity like a ballgame or some other leisure activity before or afterward?

- Does the person you will be sharing time with have any diet restrictions or other requirements?

- Does the person need help to eat? How much?

- Does the person have difficulty with certain foods? If so, can you have a meal that avoids the problem foods?

- Does the person require any sort of specialized equipment to help with eating? If so, do you know how to assist with these tools or will you need to help?

- Do you need some training ahead of time? Who will you contact about this?

Most important, ask yourself these questions:

- To be a good mealtime companion, what do I need? Not a mealtime companion for someone with a disability, but just a good mealtime companion. Period.

- How will I engage the person in a good, interesting conversation?

- How do I discover topics that we are both interested in?

- How do I present myself as open and willing to get to know this person better, especially if communication is difficult or unfamiliar at first?

- If the person I'm getting to know doesn't speak or requires assistance that is outside my experience, how can I handle myself to make it a rich experience for both of us?

 If you find out that an individual has swallowing difficulties, a powder additive, available for purchase in some grocery stores and pharmacies, can be added by spoonfuls to liquid to make it easier to swallow. It can be used with any liquid and can be taken anywhere. If you are at a restaurant and don't want to draw undue attention to the can, take a small bit in a discreet plastic bag. Add it to anything and tell anyone who asks that it is protein powder or a strength supplement!

Think of getting to know this person as an investment. Don't expect some instant soulmate or a mind-melding connection. This doesn't generally happen with anyone immediately, so expect that building a relationship with someone or helping an already established relationship to grow will take nurturance and patience, just like it would with anyone.

And please don't fall into that patronizing cliché of saying you understand and connect with someone who has a disability because "after all, we all have disabilities."

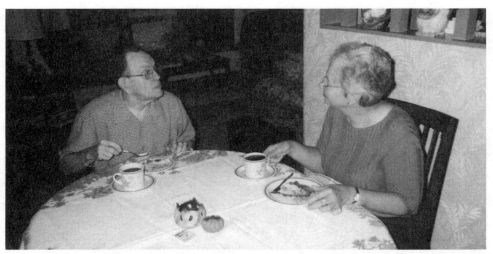

What's better than pie? Mary met Tom when he was in the state hospital in Minnesota; Mary was the librarian. "We began by celebrating our birthdays with cake and coffee. After Tom moved to a small home, we meet several times each year. Our get-togethers always include food. Tom is good company and sitting at the table gives us time to talk about things. He tells me about changes in town and about people we both know. He keeps me connected to my career and the people who are special to me. I never consider myself Tom's 'volunteer,' just his friend."

Do not demean or diminish the experiences and struggles faced by someone with a disability by comparing their life experience with yours because you wear eyeglasses or you can't reconfigure your hard drive. Do we say these things to make the other person feel more welcome and included or ourselves feel less shamed and embarrassed? After all, we don't use that same cliché when talking about the experiences of people who are of a different sexual orientation or race. Respect the significant impact a disability has on someone's life and that the person must—every day of his life—cope with all of the associated attitudes and prejudices that go with it. Try to see the world from that person's perspective, but don't co-opt it.

People who come into a relationship with a person who has a disability expecting to have some "special experience" tend to be disappointed. It's not fair to put someone on a pedestal simply because they have a disability; it's hard for anyone to live up to such high ideals. Don't try to be a special friend, just a regular one. Most people with disabilities need minimal or no extra support to share in mealtime activities. Many people who have grown up included and involved with families, friends, and in the community have learned how to participate and contribute to social situations. Others may have limited social experience or spend most of their leisure and work time with other people who have disabilities. You can model what it means to be a good friend. Remember, you are equal partners in the relationship; sometimes that may mean letting your new friend take the lead from time to time. Don't automatically plunge ahead to take care of everything. Let the person watch, learn, and try new things, such as growing something in a garden, ordering for herself in the restaurant, asking for help in the grocery store, or rolling out the pastry dough.

The grocery store, farmer's market, and flower shop are all treasure troves of sensory experiences. Take time to savor the sights, sounds, smells, and textures. Make it a hands-on experience.

If you're planning to share a meal with someone who needs partial or complete assistance to eat and you don't feel comfortable in that role, it's okay to ask someone else along, at least to get you started. A family member or a personal assistant who knows the person and does this more frequently can help you reach a comfort level with what is required. Make sure this arrangement is all right with the person who has a disability, however. After some time, you may feel more comfortable helping the person to eat. In the meantime, dinner for three can be as much fun as dinner for two. Be careful, though, not to fall into separate side conversations that leave out the person with a disability.

If you are looking for an accessible restaurant in your area, try a web search. Type in "accessible dining" and the name of your city. It will pull up a varied list of places and their accessibility features reviewed by people with disabilities.

Turn off the cell phone and television for mealtimes.

Mealtime Villains

For people who do need assistance actually getting food into their mouths during mealtime, remember you are "assuming the role of the person's hand" (J. Zgola, personal communication, 2003). As you take on that role—or while you are getting more comfortable as you learn what it involves—here are some "villains" you really must remember to avoid:

- The front-end loader—too much on the spoon
- The parachute—swooping down from above to the person's mouth
- The scraper—scraping excess food off the person's lips
- The dental assistant—wiping the mouth with the person's bib
- The helicopter—hovering the spoon in front of the person's face while he or she is chewing and swallowing the first mouthful
- Bob Barker's curtain—the person has no idea what is on the spoon but we expect him or her to take it (Zgola & Bordillon, 2001, p. 139)

Party Favors

Andrea loved to go to birthday parties to be with the other children, but the food scared him. He would see the big table with all of the things set out and he would just press himself up against the wall and he was worried people would force him to eat. He would drink things, but he just wasn't sure if other people would make him eat what he did not want. We would talk to the parents before and tell them it was okay, Andrea did not have to eat. So it was okay and not a big deal, you know? —Edi Cecchini, Italy

We know that every meal can't be perfect. People have busy lives. Details intervene. The unexpected happens. But sharing food together can remind us to pay attention to the needs of others. Not all of those needs are met merely by what's presented on our plates. Robert Perske reflects:

> When I think back all those years to what happened in the institution, I feel bad because we did things to people that sure weren't very pleasant. Sometimes we probably got more food in the lungs than we did in anybody's stomach. We probably didn't think about this then, but it's important to say now. For God's sakes, relax. Relax and just be two human beings together. Two people both having value. All right, so if someone has a severe disability, there are ways he can't contribute in certain departments but that doesn't rule out me valuing him. Through something as simple as food, well, that's the point. It's a simple way to just be with somebody.

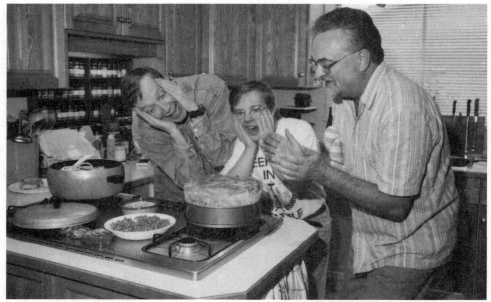

Sharing in the preparation and celebration of an unusual dish like this timpano can be the focal point of many dining experiences.

After-School Treat

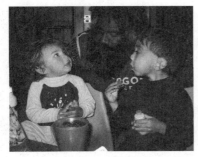

The Wylo boys have a biccie and coffee after kindy class in the afternoon and go over the day with Dad Goomblar at home in Katoomba.

Murrandah and Burung share a little wee table since they're the two young ones. It's good for Murrandah to see Burung eat and he can watch him and learn like he did with the toilet training. He enjoys his meals. I think part of it is us being all together. Teatime is the main meal, and we all sit down with the two young ones at their table. They're very close together, the young fellas, and eating is about the only time they're not fighting. He's only choked a couple of times. Green frogs are the worst because they get stuck up there. Not real green frogs, I mean the lollies.* When Murrandah and Burung come home from kindy and preschool, they generally have their usual cup of coffee. They sit at their table and dip their biccies** in coffee. It's something they look forward to every day. We teach them manners, you know, like what do you say? You say, "Thanks, mate," when you get your coffee. —Goomblar Wylo, Australia

 *candies
**cookies

Me and Me Mate'll Have a Beer

Stan was a good fella, a happy sort of bloke, and he liked having a beer. I reckon he liked going to the pub and feeling like he fit in with everyone. So from time to time, I'd take him down to the local pub, maybe after the movies or something. He'd walk up to the bar—he was only five foot nothing and about 13 stone*, a bit of a weight problem Stan had. He'd say, 'I'll have a pony.' That was a small drink, only 5 ounces. 'And a midi** for Lully,' he'd say. Used to call me Lully, always did, never Rod or Rodney, don't know why. He'd order and then he'd pay for it. I reckon he thought that was a real go, to order a beer and pay for it yourself and then stand around and talk to all the other blokes. A real man thing to do. —Rod Hall, Australia

 *182 pounds (1 stone = 14 pounds)
**midi, a drink of about 12 ounces

Pitching in, Spending Time

In Form One and Form Two*, the students did woodworking and cooking. Each student had a little book with recipes in it, and in Duncan's, the teacher went through and changed them so he could use the microwave. He just couldn't manage the oven door, so they got a little table and put a microwave on it. He was still expected to be there and do the cooking. His favorite thing was a chocolate fudge pudding (see p. 232), and he'd make that from time to time at home. In our house then, it wasn't really set up with an accessible kitchen so we had to compromise. Quite often, if I was going to do pikelets** or cake for morning tea, Duncan would come in and read the recipe for me. He'd not do so much of the actual cooking, but then none of the boys did really. So how great is this? I love cooking, but I hate running back and forth to the book, checking if I've got the measuring right. Was that a half cup or a quarter? Duncan could just read for me and we both enjoyed the time together. —Kaye Pollock, Australia

*Form 1 and 2 students range in age from 11 to 13
**small pancakes, often topped with jam and whipped cream

Does someone not have the hand strength or grasp to manage slicing cheese? Some cutting boards come with spikes to stabilize food while cutting without the need to use both hands.

Having trouble making bread "stay still" while you're making sandwiches or dressing up toast in the morning? Breadboards come with corner guards so the bread can be secured in the corner and it won't slide around.

Let's Play a Game

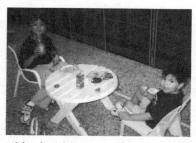

Michael and Daniel enjoy an outdoor impromptu picnic at their home in Florida.

I'm on a mission to get Danny to try new foods. Usually, if I'm hoping to get him to eat something new, I won't offer it as a choice between it and something I know he likes. I just offer the new thing. It's not really a choice if I offer something he's never tried and something he likes and I expect him to try the new thing. He won't. It might take awhile, but he'll try it if I just offer the new. Sometimes we make a game of it. I think if people saw us eating sometimes, they'd think we were all crazy. When I want him to try peas, Michael and I will feed each other one pea at a time and encourage Danny to feed us, too. He'll finally pick up the peas and feed them to us. He came very close to taking his turn to eat one. It's a game he enjoys, so maybe soon he'll try one himself. —Leigh Chou, United States

A one-handed rocker knife or ulu makes for easier cutting. No need to saw.

Comfort Food = Serenity

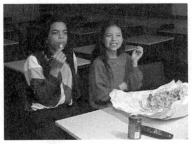

New Zealand siblings Kahurangi (left) and Harikoa share a favorite food: hot chips.

School was very stressful for Kahurangi, and that's certainly related to [the fact that he has] Asperger's syndrome. We found that the best thing we could do for him after school was to get some hot chips into him. If we could do that immediately, life had an odds-on chance of being fine for the rest of the evening. If not, there was bound to be a tantrum. We discovered that instant carbohydrates, preferably warm (hence the hot chips), were the magic wand. Luckily, there are fish and chips shops everywhere. He became very interested in comparing hot chips from different shops. He had his favorites, which I was pleased about, because it was a very small slice of life he was prepared to experiment with. And if it turned out we were having something very scary like macaroni and cheese for evening tea and he wouldn't eat it, I wasn't concerned that he was going to collapse from malnutrition. We fought the balanced diet thing for so long until we finally realized food had the potential of ruining our lives three times a day because I was trying to force Kahurangi to eat when and what he didn't want. —Bronwyn Thurlow, New Zealand

Feeling Useful

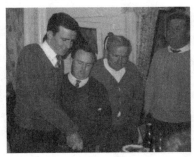

Rod, left, with brother Stan, Dad Charles and brother-in-law Neville on Rod's 21st birthday, a big occasion in Australia.

Morning and afternoon tea was generally biscuits and cakes, and Stan was right into it. Later on in life after me Dad died, when it was just Stan and Mum by themselves, he'd put the jug on and make the morning and afternoon tea. He'd time it by train time. Whenever the train would go past, that was his signal to get the tea going. The train schedule was such that they'd go out at 11 in the morning and would be back again at 3. He'd get up, boil the jug, and make the tea for him and Mum and get it all on the table. That was his little job. He thought it was quite important and it gave him something to think about. Mum let him do the washing up, too, so he felt like he was helping out. A bloke's got to feel useful, doesn't he? He could still do that with getting the tea on for Mum after his stroke, but there were many other things he wasn't sure about what he was doing after that. Mum was 81 by then and Stan was 44 when he died. When we hear the train, we still think of Stan putting on the jug. —Rod Hall, Australia

Weighted utensils and cutlery make it easier for someone with limited hand control or tremors.

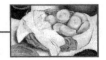

CHAPTER 10

Celebrating the Sacred in Shared Meals

Grace and Blessing

BILL GAVENTA

"Will someone say grace?"

"Who will ask the blessing?"

"Give us this day our daily bread."

So many of us open our meals with such requests. Though short and simple, they allow us to open the meal and our hearts and speak to the sacred depth and dimension of shared meals and food, both in spiritual and religious traditions, and simply in the common act of breaking bread together. Whether done in the form of a prayer, the blessing, a toast, an invocation, a song, or an invitation to come to the table, "saying grace" is a recognition that we give thanks for both the gifts of God and gifts of the earth and the work of human hands that make the meal possible. It is recognition of dependency and interdependency in the miracle of growth, the hard work of others, and the very gifts needed to sustain life.

> *"For that which we are about to receive, we give thanks."*
>
> *"Barukh attah Adonai Eloheinu Melekh ha-olam ha-motzi lehem min har-aretz."* (Blessed are You, Lord God, King of the Universe, for giving us bread, Hebrew)
>
> *"Bism Allah Al-Rahman Al-Raheem."* (In the name of God, most Gracious, most Merciful) *or* "Al-Hamdulillah" (Praise Allah) (both Arabic).

To ask the blessing is a recognition of what makes the meal possible, but it is also an action that looks forward and recognizes mutual contribution. "Bless this food, and this time together," is a way to express gratitude to God for our lives and the life of our community, whether that is family, congregation, community, culture, or country.

Those simple questions and traditions are but two small, though powerful indications of the spiritual dimensions of breaking bread together. Yet asking the blessing or saying grace probably does not happen in many residential settings in which many people with disabilities reside, perhaps because of religious diversity or misunderstandings of church/state separation. So what do you do as a parent, friend, family, advocate, or support provider when you run into people or practices that seem to exclude people with developmental disabilities from participating in a practice that may be at the heart of a faith community or religious tradition? A discussion with everyone—residents, families, and staff—might lead to ways that a group could develop their own ritual for giving thanks for the food they have, and the blessings of the day.

The traditions just described point to the central role that food and shared meals have in religious traditions and practice, as an act of community and as a sign, symbol, or sacrament of the holy in human life. The acts of sharing meals play at least three central roles.

First, think of the amazing diversity, yet common importance, in the routines and rituals of eating together in religious traditions. Think of the sacrament of Communion in Christianity, the Shabbat meal and Passover in Judaism, and the feast of the Ramadan in Islam. Or, for many congregations, a church night supper or potluck is one of the favorite congregational activities. Everyone can play a role and participate: set up, clean up, bring a dish, and share. Another sharing opportunity is the popular coffee hour after the service. A residential staff person once asked me about taking people to church, saying that she wondered why they went, because it seemed like they only went because of the coffee hour. My reply was that it was the same for lots of people! The coffee hour is where you can catch up with others, ask about what's going on, meet new people, and talk about the week ahead.

Second, religious feasts and celebrations play central roles in shaping traditions in cultural communities. What do you have to eat, in your cultural and religious background, for a particular holiday or season to be true to your tradition? Christmas, Thanksgiving, Passover, and so on would not be right without _____. You fill in the blank, in terms of food, or particular rituals of breaking bread together. Asking staff, families, and people with disabilities to bring those favorite dishes to a holiday celebration is not only great eating but also a celebration of cultural and religious diversity.

Third, in addition to seasonal rituals, think of the role that food plays in building and celebrating community at various times of an individual's life cycle. To name but a few, there is wafer given during the First Communion, the cake at a birthday party, the party after a bar or bat mitzvah or a wedding, and the cross-cultural traditions of bringing food to friends at times of crisis, death, and grief.

One of the most common struggles in many group homes and residential settings is what to do after someone dies. Why not put the word out that people could bring food, like they do everywhere else, and thus facilitate times of eating, remembering, grieving, and loving together? Or, residents of one home could be encouraged to work together to prepare a dish or a plate of cookies for friends in another home if someone has died.

The spiritual dimensions of shared food and drink are thus as diverse as they are deep. Sharing food can be an act of hospitality, an act of gratitude, an act of remembrance, an act of celebration of the present, and an act that looks forward to the possibilities of life or what community can be. Shared food and religious rituals that incarnate that sharing become ways of affirming and recognizing that which sustains, renews, heals, and blesses. The old Western saying, "The way to a man's heart is through his stomach" could simply be modified: "To understand the heart of a particular faith tradition, look at the rituals involving food and breaking bread together."

Early in my career, a young minister taking a course on ministries with people with disabilities relayed an experience from her congregation. Several people from a local group home had come to communion for the first time. Afterward, in the coffee hour, the young minister went over to their table, noting that they seemed to be very excited and happy. The following conversation ensued:

Minister:	You seem happy and excited today.
Visitor from a group home:	Yeah, I ate with you in church today.
Minister:	Yes, do you know what that is called?
Visitor:	No, you tell me.
Minister:	It is called communion. We do this because of what happened to Jesus, when he ate supper before he died . . . (and she went on to try to explain the significance.)
Visitor:	No, No. Don't tell me that. Tell me the part about all of us doing it together. I ate with you in church today!

Thus, to be included, or to partake, in those traditions and rituals, is to be included in the heart of community and, to some, in the heart of one's higher being. And to be excluded from a tradition or ritual because of a developmental disability or some other issue is to be separated in ways that can be extremely painful. One of my first teachers was a Catholic mother who, in telling about the experience of having her son denied first communion, said, "When he [the priest] rejected my son, he rejected me." Conversely, the experiences of being included in communion or in other religious rituals that involve breaking bread together become powerful experiences of affirmation and expressions of community. Community, for everyone, is strengthened. Hospitality to the stranger, in acts that involve sharing food, is at the heart of so many faith traditions.

Here are some ideas for transforming barriers into opportunities and possibilities:

- *Recognize that resistance may simply reflect hesitancy, uncertainty, and anxiety that comes from something new—a fear and the desire to protect what one holds most dearly (e.g., a sense of holiness).* A pastor, priest, or rabbi may simply have never done this before. Blend a recognition of their desire to protect the holy or what is most special with helping them to see why this may be so special for the person or family involved and how it could be a special moment for the whole congregation.

- *Come with stories and examples from other congregations within a given tradition who have done just that.* There are many positive and powerful stories out there. Find some, and put those clergy in touch with others in their tradition who can serve as a guide and resource. Every major faith tradition has examples of people with multiple and severe disabilities being included in rituals such as communion and bar/bat mitzvahs.

- *Get the doctrine right.* Sometimes exclusion comes from misunderstandings, or old understandings, of doctrine or practice within a given tradition.

- *Learn how to do what for me is a fundamental skill in community building: Reverse the question.* When someone asks, "How do we know this person will understand the significance of the sacrament or ritual?" a clergy person might respond, "How do we know *anyone* does?" If people are to be excluded for incomplete understanding or their own weaknesses, then that would exclude most everyone. But reverse it with understanding, and use this as an opportunity for saying that you also want them to learn as much as they are capable about the significance of the act, and that you have some ideas for how to do that.

- Recognize that the *training, education, or learning* that can take place before participation in a sacrament or ritual can be a way of *building new relationships and community connections* that could lead, in fact, to ongoing friendships.

- Finally, make sure that as you work on inclusion within religious and spiritual practices, traditions, and communities, you *focus on the gifts people bring and the ways they can and do bless others.* Or, stated another way, focus on contributions that people with disabilities can make to the shared meals of faith communities. That can mean helping out at the church night supper with set up or clean up; working with the residents of a group home to make and bring a dish to the supper or to someone within the congregation who is in need or crisis; or inviting the pastor, priest, or rabbi to the home for coffee, a meal, or a picnic.

The question is not just how people with disabilities are invited and welcomed into the rituals of faith communities, but how they, as well, can invite and contribute. They are not just "consumers" of meals or community prepared by others, but in fact they can and do serve as channels of grace and agents of blessings to others.

 In western countries, there are interfaith, ecumenical, and specific faith networks that connect people who are committed to inclusion of people with disabilities and their families. Those include the Religion and Spirituality Division of the AAMR, the Christian Council for Persons with Disabilities, the National Apostolate for Inclusion Ministries, the National Catholic Partnership with People with Disabilities, and the Religion and Disability Program of the National Organization on Disability.

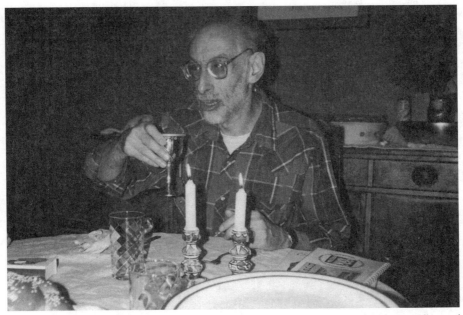

Mel of Toronto celebrates Shabbat in his L'Arche home. He has just lit the Shabbat candles and is going to say the blessing for the wine after reviewing the blessings in a Reena Foundation booklet that gives syllabic and English translations. Mel has his own kiddish cup and other ceremonial items. He was proud to have his Bar Mitzvah at the age of 54.

Keeping the Faith

Shabbat has become an important tradition in Mel Kirzner's house. Mel celebrates Shabbat on Friday evenings with his L'Arche* house members, lighting the candles, saying the blessings for the wine and challah, and enjoying a special meal. Others in his house are not Jewish, but enjoy sharing the Shabbat meal with Mel. Mel has a booklet with the Hebrew blessings in syllabics so that an assistant can read them aloud with him. This is important in enabling Mel to celebrate this central Jewish tradition because although Mel knows the blessings fairly well, he is legally blind and is not quite confident enough to say them alone.

Ending a meal with prayer is a Jewish tradition and also one practiced by L'Arche. Mel and his housemates end their meals by reciting the 23rd Psalm instead of the Lord's Prayer, used in most L'Arche communities, or the traditional Jewish Grace After Meals, which is in Hebrew and would be quite difficult for all to say. They began this custom after Mel's father died and Mel was saying Kaddish. One of the assistants noted that Psalm 23 featured prominently in the little book of prayers Mel was given by the Jewish funeral home.

Each year, a community pre-Passover seder is led by Ellen Weinstein's parents and friends from the synagogue where Ellen, another L'Arche member, and Mel attend. It's a very popular event, a wonderful celebration, and a good educational

*L'Arche is an international network of faith-based communities for people with developmental disabilities and those who assist them. Now at 130 communities on 5 continents, it was created by Jean Vanier in France in 1964.

opportunity for all of us who are not Jewish. When we have a Friday evening service for Shabbat, we act out the welcoming of the Shabbat Queen. Ellen enters wearing a white shawl over her head and shoulders, looking a bit like a bride, while we sing the song welcoming Shabbat, L'ha Dodi. The service is made simple and accessible in other ways, too. We don't use much Hebrew and what we do use is translated. There is a little sermon or simple and memorable reflection in story form from the rabbis. —Beth Porter, Canada

---

 Wondering about mealtimes in different religions and faiths? Visit http://www.familyvillage.wisc.edu/, and click on House of Worship, which has related resources, materials, and organizations. Also try http://www.qualitymall.org and the Religion and Spirituality Division, AAMR at: http://www.aamrreligion.org.

Appreciating the Ritual

Jim and I aren't regulars at church . . . truth be told, we're barely irregular. But last summer we went, and it was a service that included communion. Jim had taken communion a few times when he was younger, but neither of us had ever done it at this church, or in recent memory. So I kind of studied what everyone was doing ahead of us (yes, we were in a back pew), and I whispered some hurried instructions to Jim. He nodded, but I had the distinct sense that he was humoring me. "Yeh, sure Dad, I get it." So I was just hoping he'd do everything right when it was showtime.

The ushers invited our pew to come up. We joined the pre-communion line-up in the center aisle of the church and did our best to look contemplative. Actually, Jim did that much better than I did, because I was more concerned about what he was doing than I was with what I should have been doing. We eased ourselves into position and knelt at the railing, and Jim was just perfect—hands folded, head bowed (but all the while checking me out of the corner of his eye). When the minister came up, Jim held out his hand and accepted the host and popped it in his mouth. "Mmmmmmm" I heard him exclaim, "good." I threw him *the look*. He got it, but looked confused. I could tell he was thinking: "It's never a problem when Karin, Dad, and I have our evening wine and cheese." Oh no . . . wine and cheese! Then came the wine, and I knew, just knew, what was about to follow. He knocked back the tiny challis and announced, "Cheers!"

As we were walking back to our seats, me sheepishly and Jim happily, I noticed that almost everyone we passed was smiling and nodding to Jim. They weren't the least bit bothered—in fact, they seemed to see something that completely eluded me in my cloud of embarrassment. He was happy—really happy—and communion is a celebration of faith, after all. Jim got it right, and he showed me a lot that day about what it means to be devout. —Richard Schwier, Canada

CHAPTER 11

The Social Implications of Mealtime

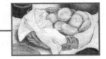

The gentle art of gastronomy is a friendly one.
It hurdles the language barrier,
makes friends among civilized people,
and warms the heart.
—SAMUEL CHAMBERLAIN (AS CITED IN THE SWIVEL COLLECTIVE, 2002)

Mealtime typically presents daily opportunities for people with disabilities to feel productive, responsible, and in control over some portion of their activities. Decisions around the time for a meal, grocery shopping, food selection, preparation, and consumption are all chances for choice, participation, and enjoyable interaction with others.

When most people think about eating, favorite foods come to mind, along with the family and friends they like to share these foods with and the places where they like to eat them. Worth is placed on mealtime not only for nutritional value but also for the interaction it promotes.

Whether it's a barbecue with friends, Dad's waffles on Sunday mornings, or dinner out on Tuesday, people place their unique social and emotional values on dining experiences and, at the same time, benefit from the social aspects of dining with others. Unless we are all alone on a deserted island, gnawing on a coconut, mealtimes have vast potential for social experiences. Even a solitary mealtime in a restaurant provides opportunities for conversations with servers and, perhaps, even with other diners.

In historic hunting and gathering cultures, mealtime involved the task of getting adequate nutrients to one's family. Stripped to their most fundamental purposes,

Remember what you enjoy at mealtime: easy conversation, good humor, nice music, a calm atmosphere, and tasty food. Some people with disabilities may take some time to see this as a pleasant alternative to the rushed, noisy, overstimulated, staff-driven experience they may be used to having.

hunting and gathering validated a person's role and status, desire to participate, and concept of self-worth. Today, adequately feeding the family and one's friends still contributes to someone's sense of accomplishment and self-esteem. It's a liberating experience. Even people who claim, "I can't cook," find a sense of value and identity in telling the tales of kitchen mishaps and disasters. They are still comforted by an image of themselves in the kitchen and find an identity and empathy with others who say, "I don't make dinner. I make reservations."

Today, the people who grow food, harvest it, inspect it, package it, ship it, sell it, cook it, serve it, and clean it up are members of a vast array of honorable professions in the farming and food service industry. Mealtimes, then, whether one is creating them one's self or asking someone else to provide them, are experiences valued on multiple levels that lend validity to everyone involved. However, this opportunity for affirmation is so often denied to people with disabilities.

NOURISHING MEMBERSHIP AND FELLOWSHIP

Mealtime can provide a rich environment for growth and discovery. It can embrace and welcome people who need community, and it can support their capacity to contribute. The secret is often in how others offer that support and opportunity.

How do actions and interactions (and those of others) represent the person with a disability? Is the message being conveyed that this person is someone to be with or someone to take care of? Be aware—and beware—of the subtle signals that may be sent without one realizing it. These signals can be negative, such as when a person with a disability sits silently at a table while others talk around him instead of to him, or positive, as in this example:

Coming out of a small neighborhood restaurant one evening, a young man with Down syndrome holds the door for his parents. As he steps onto the sidewalk, he offers his arm to his mother. In the other hand, he carefully carries a white Styrofoam box with a few choice leftovers. The family, animated in conversation about the meal, moves off toward their car. Unknown to them, a young couple sits at an nearby outdoor table, consoling themselves with tea and reeling over their newborn's diagnosis of Down syndrome. They have recently emigrated to Canada from England, know only a handful of people, and find themselves overwhelmed with confusion and grief.

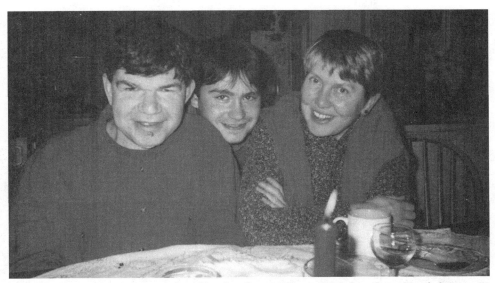

Mike, Christian, and Beth linger at the table after dinner. Mike and Beth have been friends for over 20 years and once lived in the same L'Arche home. Christian came from Germany to spend two years in L'Arche.

Dee Cole, the young mother, said later:

> *I can't really explain why watching that family had such a powerful effect on us, but in those few seconds, our despair turned into hope for our daughter's future. They were just a family, out for supper, and their son seemed like such a considerate person. It just looked so ordinary. We sat there in tears, but for the first time in days, we could laugh.*

We are reminded of the ingenious invisibility cloak worn by Harry Potter in J.K. Rowling's novels. Harry was able to wrap himself in the cloak and become completely invisible. As we stand beside a person with a disability, it begs the questions: Do we cloak her as less than competent, less than equal, as someone to be looked after, even pitied? Are we embarrassed or uncomfortable so much that we allow her to fade away? Do we speak to and interact with that person in a way that is different from how we interact with others? Do we make the person with a disability disappear by simply doing everything for her while expecting no contribution from her in return?

Fully including someone with a disability means more than just talking to the person during mealtimes. It may also mean holding that person to some of the same standards of etiquette as would be expected of anyone. In Canada, the 60-year-old brother of a 52-year-old man with Down syndrome laments the lack of table manners taught at his brother's group home. "Appalling" is the word the older brother uses to describe his younger sibling's behavior at the table. He wonders why he can't consume a meal like a "civilized human being." Sadly, visits between the siblings that involve a family sit-down meal are rare because "he really makes everyone lose their appetites."

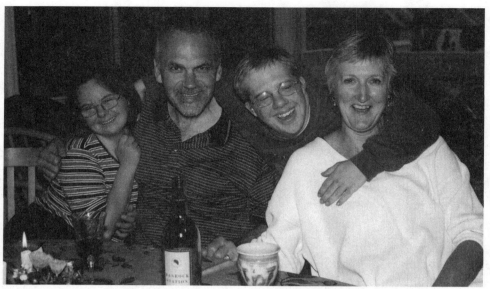

Friends Liz, Al, Jim, and Vickie (left to right) strike an after-dinner pose.

The younger brother has only a moderate disability and seems to look after his other personal needs such as hygiene and dressing. "I don't know why they can't teach him some table manners," the brother adds.

Why indeed. This institutional eating behavior—bolting food; grabbing; chewing open-mouthed; and failing to use utensils, serviettes, or napkins properly—is clearly an example of living in an environment in which residents are fed rather than dine together or share a meal. The cloak of incompetence tightly wrapped around this man's brother is keeping him apart from family and potential friends.

Instead, why not wrap someone in a cloak of competence—transparent enough that the light can shine in on the individual's value, worth, gifts, and abilities? Are we confident and secure enough to take a step back and let the individual offer her unique gifts and contributions? Does the cloak rest lightly enough on his shoulders that he can simply be a fellow human being? Can it still be snug enough to provide warmth and security while he learns the skills he needs to make his journey? One of the best ways a person can show off skills to others is through mealtimes. Learning the various tasks and skills associated with planning, cooking, preparing, and sharing meals go a long way toward making someone feel "visible."

 Are people living in the home encouraged to clear after a meal? Many people feel proud to help tidy up. Always be ready with compliments and thanks for the help. Everyone needs to feel like they are doing for themselves.

Do people know how to use the microwave? A simple chart with a food item and the time for cooking or warming up can be an easy guide to kitchen independence.

People rarely feel alone and isolated around the table or in a warm, fragrant kitchen. Taking time to enjoy and experience the moments of mealtime, before, during, and after the meal itself can create a sense of calm and belonging that promotes value and worth. We can nourish a sense of security and welcome by being mindful and aware of mealtimes together.

Providing a time not only for the enjoyment of the food itself but also for one another's company can create comfortable connections to be appreciated both by those participating in the meal and by those observing.

In this connectedness, participants are shown an example of what is possible. For many, like Dee Cole, it might provide a glimpse of something that transcends the old myths and stereotypes about people with disabilities.

Are people welcome in the kitchen? One residential director we know makes it a practice to invite people into the kitchen to help with muffins and cookies. If they don't feel like helping, they might enjoy a cup of tea or coffee, and it's visiting time while the kitchen is warm and wonderful with baking.

Community and Growth

Author Jean Vanier spoke about the role of food and mealtimes in spiritual growth:

> Human beings need bread if they are to grow. If they don't eat, they die. And if they are to grow spiritually, they, like plants, need sun, water, air and soil. The soil is community—the place where they are planted, take root, grow, give fruit and die so that others may live. (1989, p. 165)

He also noted,

> When a mother feeds her baby, there is mutual presence, joy and play. An infant who is not fed with love and who takes the nipple mechanically is going to have indigestion. Human beings don't eat like animals, all in their own corner. Friendship and love make the activity human. . . . This is why meals must not be times for contentious discussion or serious educational attitudes. Working meals are not to be encouraged either. A meal is a time of relaxation for the body and the spirit. Laughter is excellent for the digestion. Serious discussions cause ulcers and other intestinal problems. Some children really do have terrible problems if they can't eat in an atmosphere of relaxation. I know that tensions at the table cut my appetite and go straight to my liver! . . . . We have a duty to learn more cre-

ative ways of celebrating. We need to find more rousing and funnier songs, stories, and snippets of information. If these can be well prepared, the meal and other community activities can become moments of sharing, celebration and pooling of knowledge, with all the opening of spirit that these imply. Too many people come to a meal simply as consumers. They don't realize the role which meals can play in the building of community. (Vanier, 1989, pp. 322–324)

We Gather Together: Ideas for Sharing Food Preparation

Mealtime lends itself to so many festive group experiences; Italian dishes especially lend themselves to cooperative preparation. Lasagna, cannelloni, manicotti, pizza, and calzones all require lots of chopping, stuffing, and layering—tasks that are fun to do together. Homemade pizza can be a fun joint project. Make a homemade or use store-bought crust. Spread with tomato sauce, and then the sky's the limit on toppings. You can even fold the whole thing over in the end to make a big calzone.

Of course, foods from other cultures are great for get-togethers, too. Tamales are perfect for making in large quantities at one time. Families, community organizations, and churches will gather and start an assembly line to make 24 dozen or more in one go to either fill freezers, feed a throng during a big celebration or in response to a community crisis, or sell at a local farmers market or street fair. Shishkebabs are a good dish for sharing preparation tasks. Marinate cubes of meat in teriyaki sauce—or your own marinade. Soak wooden skewers in water for one half hour. Cut vegetables such as zucchini; onion; and green, red, and yellow peppers in large pieces to match the size of the meat. Use whole mushrooms. Tomatoes don't stand up well to the heat, so put them on after grilling. Cherry or grape tomatoes work well. People can have fun assembling their own kebabs before putting them on the barbeque.

Try juicing. It makes for a fun afternoon of chopping up apples, carrots, ginger, limes, and lemons in chunks (and you can do it on the cheap by finding fruit that may be just past its prime—not too much past!). Someone with limited fine motor skills can still manage to drop the chunks into the machine, and the results are immediate!

 When making food with large groups, split the tasks. If making an entire pie or four dozen cookies is too much for one session, try mixing the ingredients on one occasion. Pop the dough in the freezer. Thaw the dough in preparation for the next time you get together.

Pre-prepare and package meals in separate containers; store in the refrigerator or freezer and with reheating instructions. This can make for easy and more independent cooking.

Music, Food, and Smiles

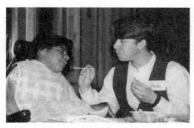

Alia (left), who is Muslim, and friend Sheilagh. Sheilagh once lived with Alia in a L'Arche home and is now an Anglican priest. At an interfaith seder, Alia enjoys tasting various foods with a sponge stick, but takes her actual nutrition through a tube.

We work at ways to include Alia and recognize her Muslim faith identity, inviting Muslim friends and Alia's family to help us. While Alia cannot speak or see, she responds with a happy smile to rhythm and to hearing Arabic chanted. We have tapes of Arabic songs that she enjoys and encourage those close to Alia to learn the Muslim greeting of peace. At Eid*, we all shared a special dessert made by a Muslim friend. —Beth Porter, Canada

*Eid-ul-Fitr is a celebratory feast at the end of Ramadan, the Muslim holy month of fasting.

Anticipation is more than half the fun of a meal. Do you plan for Thanksgiving feast the day before? Chances are, you're thinking about it for at least weeks ahead of time. Help someone with a disability enjoy the flood of feelings and sensations that lead up to your time together.

Pass the Understanding, Please

Things have been rough lately around here. Since the beginning of November, Dave has had a lot of seizures. He's had two bad falls, and one left him unable to walk or stand for several days, though it was neat to see him get up and start walking again on Christmas day. Like our own little Tiny Tim. Anyway, Dave had a nasty strep infection and then some kind of flu. We've been to the emergency departments in Edmonton and Vancouver as well as a bunch of doctor visits. So our life, which has always been in a shambles, has reached a state of disorganization in which we can only hope to achieve shambles with a lot of hard work and a little luck. David's seizures now involve a lot of yelling at the top of his lungs and a lot of gagging at the end, which often ends in vomiting. Last night we cleared out Burger King in less than 1 minute. —Dick Sobsey, Canada

A Place at the Table to the End

When I was living in the L'Arche home in Calgary, there was a [man] in his early seventies. He had Down syndrome. I didn't know it then, but he was dying. He was getting 24-hour nursing care. Social Services in Alberta informed the people that this man was ready to go into a nursing home. The L'Arche people said, "No, he isn't. He's been living here for 22 years, and he's going to die in his home." So they made an arrangement for nursing care and someone would check on him a couple of times during the night. They massaged his feet and his hands with oil and made things so good for him. There was no question that he would come to table for mealtime. When he came to table, he would sit in a reclining chair and one of the women would help him. At breakfast, he ate two eggs and two pieces of toast. All the while, there were great rattles in his lungs as if he was going to die any second. But they treated him so gently. They'd touch his face and smile at him and he'd smile back. Seven weeks later, he passed away. But he passed away surrounded by those he loved. There are still pictures all over the house of him in healthier times with his cowboy hat on. He was a real joker, a real nice guy, and one of the founding members of that home. There are all kinds of stories that will go on forever because people will never forget him. —Robert Sanche, Canada

What David, his family, the man with Down syndrome in the L'Arche home, and so many others yearn for—and bask in when it happens—is that climate of belonging in community, whether it be around one's own table at home or at a neighborhood restaurant. When the feeling of being welcomed and wanted is bestowed, even when one may have habits or behaviors that are unfamiliar and sometimes even unpleasant for others, it is the best a caring community can offer. Sometimes, individuals with disabilities and their families must also assert their own right to their place in the community. In doing so, they remind others they do not want mere tolerance but equal citizenship, seizures and all.

 For someone who can scoop but can't quite turn the utensil into the mouth, there are spoons available that are angled to the right or left of the stem to point directly at the mouth. These are also easily made by picking up some lightweight utensils at your local thrift or consignment store and bending them to fit your needs.

 Cut-away cups allow the cup to be tipped up high enough without the person tipping her head back. Cut-away cups can be made from dishwasher-safe plastic. Make your own by cutting and sanding out a piece, or order from catalogues.

For people whose physical disabilities keep them from being neat eaters, how about hosting a toga party? Nobody worries about spills and messes if everybody's wearing a sheet!

Sharing Goes Both Ways

Dianne Ferguson, Ph.D., teaches at the Center on Human Development, University of Oregon in Eugene. She insists that the goal for people with disabilities is membership, that sense of belonging, and for others to embrace their inclusion:

> Satisfying, active, contributory membership depends upon fostering the kinds of interest, shared meanings, and relationships upon which socially meaningful communication must be based...membership cannot be reduced to acts, forms, functions, or repertoires. Membership cannot be predicted or controlled, it must be conferred. (1994, p. 10)

True community inclusion and welcome doesn't happen just because of billboards and awareness ads in the newspaper. It doesn't happen just because people without disabilities make an extra effort to include people with disabilities. Inclusion "at the table" goes two ways; it happens when people with disabilities make their presence known and their value felt. People without disabilities can be supportive, but welcome also happens when people with disabilities make others believe they belong.

Now and then, stop and think about what our words, attitudes, and actions say about our friends, family members, and the people we work with who have disabilities. In an effort to protect them, do we stand in the way of someone determined to make her presence felt by people who believe she doesn't belong? Or, going back to our analogy, do we offer her a cloak, lightly resting on her shoulders, so that she can change her community through her own hospitality?

Talk with someone who has a disability in the same tone of voice as you would with anyone else. Avoid the temptation to singsong or end all of your sentences in an upswing as if they are questions.

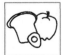

Do you remember how undignified you felt when your mom would pull an old tissue out of her purse and wipe your face in public? Or worse, when she would lick her thumb and try to scrub something off of your face? Please don't do that to anyone!

Now Andrea's Really Cool!

You know how friends are when they are together. They run around and play and then they want to stop for a break and have something to eat and to drink. This was something Andrea never wanted. "No," he would say, and it would be a nightmare for him and for me. He simply did not want to eat solid foods until he was 10 years old. The change happened very suddenly. He would always have to bring all his food and drink with him, but now he can find something he will want to try. Along with his new interest in trying foods, Andrea has also decided he will try sparkling drinks. One of his schoolmates came to me at the end of this year and he said, "I think Andrea is really cool because now he drinks Coke!" —Edi Cecchini, Italy

Try to Be a Good Chef

Kathy, Shelly, and I go grocery shopping. I make a list of what I need, what I'm out of. I get the cart and we pick up what we need. Sometimes we buy chicken, sometimes liver, sometimes pork chops. And sandwich meat, bread, and milk. And fruit for lunches, that's important, oh, you bet. And yogurt. And mixed vegetables. And chicken nuggets, the ones that are frozen in the box.

Last week I helped Kathy make a birthday cake. I used foil to cover it because plastic wrap sticks to it. I helped make chocolate cupcakes in a muffin tin. We celebrate my birthdays, especially the big party for my 60th birthday. When Kathy cooks things for the freezer, I get out the containers to pack things in the freezer. I help with the lids. We mark the containers with masking tape. Then we know what we have. When we cook, I get everything out for Kathy and I help her.

Kathy showed me how to make a grilled cheese sandwich. Put the cheese between two slices of bread, butter it, and put it in the frying pan 'til it gets brown. Flip it. Cut it in two. I learned how to fry hamburgers. Kathy made the hamburgers and I fried them until they got brown. Shelly set out the buns.

I can make a baked potato. Wash the potato. Poke it with a fork. Put it in the microwave oven for 6-0-0. I like bacon bits and sour cream on my baked potato. We make baked chicken, too. Put chicken pieces in a roaster and then add what you want. Kathy says to use what's in the pantry. Sometimes we use barbecue sauce on the chicken, sometimes Shake and Bake or cream of mushroom soup. My mom was a good cook. When I went home, she would have lunch ready. I helped clean up the dishes, I sure did. We would have a nap, and then go to McDonald's for a fresh coffee. I try to be a good chef. That's my life story. —Darlene Leister, Canada

Good Times

Sometimes Aunya and me, we goes to the Florida Panthers game, ball games, bowling sometimes. I get me some of them cheese fries. We get together 'bout two times every month. I feel real sad right there, real disappointed if we don't see each other no more. So we just keep right on doing it. I have pizza with blue cheese from Papa John's, you get some of them wings and blue cheese. That is so delicious for me! When we is eating, I tell Aunya 'bout my driving, I keep study my driving book so I pass the test. I get my moped maybe this summer or the fall and if I get more than five wrong answers, I keep taking it two, three, four times till I get it and get my license. Then I pick Aunya up. We go to the Marlins ball game and get some nachos and chili and maybe chicken tenders and fries. That's a good time. —Carl Shell, United States

When planning a shopping trip to find the ingredients for a meal to prepare together, give someone who has little or no language skills a chance to help prepare the list. Spread a sale flier out and suggest he circle some of the items you need. Take the flier along to the store and hunt down the circled items together. If a grocery shopping experience is a bit overwhelming, try a small convenience store. Or go with a list so you can contain the experience but still get out and about.

Pre-cut and washed vegetables and salad fixings are available in the produce section, or you can make your own ahead of time and store in an airtight bag. For beginning cooks, or people who want to get to the finish line more quickly, the end result is more apparent sooner. Adding extra tomatoes, zucchini, green peppers, and radishes to a bowl of ready-made salad still creates a sense of achievement quickly!

Ready to pull apart/cut-and-bake cookies, bread, pizza crust, dinner rolls, and biscuits are available in most dairy or bakery sections of the grocery store. These can offer a sense of immediate accomplishment. Cookie dough from scratch can be made ahead and frozen in portions, ready to pull out for an afternoon of baking.

Celebrating Milestones

Kahurangi is now 14. Too tall, all elbows and knees, too tall, growing like the proverbial weed, too tall, cheerfully and successfully home-schooled, too tall, still surviving mostly on baked beans and hot chips, too tall, healthy, too tall, big footed, too tall, and growing out of clothes as fast as we get him some and oh, by the way, he is too tall. Great celebrations are held when he grows taller than some of his closest adult friends. The ceremony of baking him a cake to mark this transition has sort of fallen into place within the *whanau**. As he grows taller than someone, they have to bake him a cake. It is the marking that is important. There was one cake that I don't think he did more than take a token nibble himself. It wasn't baked beans or hot chips but it is the sort of wacky, no-stress celebration symbol that can allow lots of laughter and non-competitive competition. He is very clear that there is no virtue accruing to his growing taller; but it is a social signal of sorts. —Bronwyn Thurlow, New Zealand

* extended family

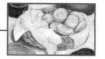

CHAPTER 12

Giving and Receiving Hospitality

The ultimate aim of civility and good manners is to please:
to please one's guest or to please one's host. To this end one uses the rules
laid down by tradition: of welcome, generosity, affability, cheerfulness, and
consideration for others. People entertain warmly and joyously. To persuade a
friend to stay for lunch is a triumph and a precious honor. To entertain many
together is to honor them all mutually. It is equally an honor to be a guest.
—CLAUDIA RODEN

Powerful words not often heard by people with disabilities are the hallmarks of hospitality: "please" and "thank you." People with disabilities are expected to say these things, but how often is *their* hospitality acknowledged? How often do people with disabilities have occasion to say, "You're welcome"? Preparing, offering, and sharing food are valued occupations of human relationships.

Think of the pride with which we offer food. How do we feel if someone comes to our home and we have nothing to offer? Even a cup of tea and a plate of cookies is a gift of hospitality we enjoy when we offer it or receive it. For many people with disabilities who live in settings in which they are "served," the idea of providing opportunities for them to control social situations in their residence is sometimes forgotten. The act of welcoming guests and providing them with food might increase the emotional and physical health of someone who lives life according to agency rules. A simple gesture of gratitude doesn't take much, but what it can do for an individual's sense of self-worth is priceless.

Consider this scene in the cozy kitchen of a group home in Saskatchewan, Canada:

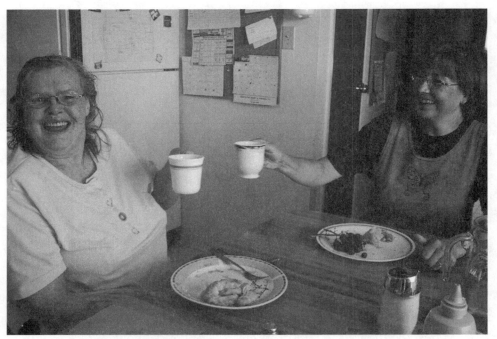

Mary and Irene toast Mary's recent bingo winnings.

"Good morning, Mary. The coffee's on. What do you feel like for breakfast this morning?"

"Coffee, coffee first, yes. Yes," says Mary, shuffling in, smoothing down gray, bed-mussed hair.

This exchange between a residential support staff and Mary, a 65-year-old woman who spent many years in an institution, gently welcomes her into the kitchen this autumn morning. Mary, who has a significant disability, shares the home with four other seniors. She helps herself to coffee and, with difficult speech, wonders aloud whether she should have her bath before or after breakfast. She settles down at the kitchen table with a cup of coffee and adds milk and sugar generously. While she sips and slowly acclimatizes to the day, a staff person chats with her about any plans she might have. After a while, a second staff person asks if she'd like her bath started, and Mary says yes. When she comes out 15 minutes later, freshly dressed and hair combed, the support staff compliments her on how good she looks. Baths have been a trial for Mary in the past. She needs assistance in the tub, and she doesn't like water in her face.

"How about a late breakfast, Mary? Would you like to come up and serve yourself or do you want me to do up a plate?"

Mary says she's not too hungry, but she'll get her own toast and another coffee.

This is a small town, so no one is surprised when the doorbell rings later and an agency board member is invited in. She's just popped over for a hello since she was at the neighborhood church.

"Stay for lunch?" Mary asks, working on her third coffee. "Sandwiches, yes, yes. Shirley makes cabbage salad."

"Well, thank you, Mary. I'd love to stay! Thanks for asking me," says Irene.

Mary beams. That someone "beams" is so often a cliché but it's the only possible way to describe Mary's face as Irene pulls up a chair at the table. When the food is ready, everyone helps themselves except for Mary, who has some difficulty walking. She asks a staff person to get her plate for her. The staff person puts the plate on the table and explains what is on it. Irene and Mary have lunch and chat at one end of the table. The other residents come in; one announces he will eat in the living room so he can watch the football game. The staff eat at the same time at the table. Mary reminds one of the staff that her son's eighth birthday is coming up (she remembers them all). She reminds Irene about bingo at the New Horizons senior's center on Wednesday. The last time she went, she won $4.50. "Coffee money," she chuckles. The kitchen is warm, animated—and ordinary.

Think of the lessons being taught in this morning scenario. Mary, who is a senior with significant disabilities, is given the dignity that older people deserve. She gets up when she wants to in the morning. People speak calmly and gently. Laughter can be heard. The staff asks Mary about her preferences and opinions. She is given support when necessary but in a subtle way that reinforces her independence. She has control. She can invite an unexpected visitor to stay for lunch, and she can entertain in her home. This morning scenario proves that services for people with disabilities don't have to feel like "services," and often the interactions that make life ordinary happen around the kitchen table.

Hospitality is a self-empowerment concept that people with disabilities can extend to one another. Rather than a group of people in a residential facility who sit and wait for staff to initiate activities and serve and support them, people with disabilities can learn to welcome each other to the table. The ideal is not that people with disabilities should be congregated only with one another, but that staff join them and share the meal. Often, when staff or caregivers have power, people with disabilities experience a feeling of resignation. The power must be shared so that mealtime can be one in which the giving and receiving of hospitality and fellowship is everyone's responsibility.

Making up a nice pot of tea and setting out a plate of cookies is an important cultural tradition and social nicety that Hoppy Sammons and Irene Lamb of Christchurch, New Zealand, relish. Both had lived in institutions for many years and, because they were friends, staff who knew them well saw that they moved together into a small supported living home in Christchurch.

> Wearing a sleeveless cotton housedress and worn slippers, Irene, 59, surveys the rickety kitchen table laden with several plates of sliced loaves and fancy biscuits. Her deeply wrinkled face, *sans* teeth, creases into a smile as Hoppy, 68, shuffles into the dining room with the kettle. Irene holds the teapot steady as Hoppy pours. (Melberg Schwier, 1994, p. 161)

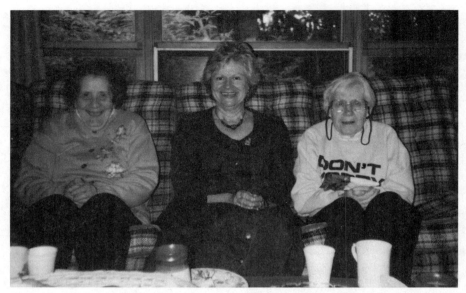

Anne, Mary Jane, and Thelus visit at a summer buffet. The three women have been friends since Mary Jane was an assistant in L'Arche in the 1970s.

When their guest asks to take a photograph of the couple, they argue over who should hold the teapot and who should hold the plate of ANZAC biscuits. Unfortunately for the photographer, the truce required that no one hold anything.

 Arrange for people living in your residential agency to invite family and friends for dinner now and then. Make sure people can show off their skills and talents in the kitchen.

Dr. Dick Sobsey is the director of the J.P. Das Developmental Disabilities Centre, University of Alberta, in Edmonton, Canada. He's also the parent of a young son with disabilities. Sobsey, a registered nurse, at one time worked in an institution in New York for people with disabilities. He recalls a memorable mealtime with one of the residents that reinforced the lesson that human beings, no matter who they are or where they're from, can connect on fundamental levels:

I was working at the Wassaic State School in New York. It was Thanksgiving, and I had to work late. Even though I was only about 50 miles from my family, it didn't make sense for me to make the trip after work. There was this guy who lived in the institution, and I offered to take him out for Thanksgiving dinner with me. What I didn't realize was that there really weren't any restaurants open, so we started driving. We kept going further and further, looking for anything open, until we finally just showed up sort of unannounced at my sister's. I didn't feel like I should just tell everybody [about the man's intellectual disabilities], so I didn't say anything. We all sat down to eat. This guy's verbal skills were not bad and he probably didn't look very different from other people I brought home. Nobody really asked where he was from. It was neat to see the interaction. Here's a guy who'd spent the last 40 years of his life in the institution, and I doubt he'd had a meal in anybody's house in all that time. It was interesting to see how little difference it made. People were chatting and sometimes I could tell he didn't have a clue, but it didn't matter. Like my brother-in-law would say, "Oh, I hate the president. He's such a jerk." And this guy would agree, "Yeah, he is a jerk!" It didn't really matter that he didn't know who the president was, but it was great to see him connect and want to reinforce on an emotional level what people were saying.

Mealtime-related opportunities to contribute and give back to the community are plentiful. Organizations such as the Salvation Army, food banks, friendship inns, soup kitchens, and community gardens are always searching for volunteers. Supporting people with disabilities to give back to their communities helps them step outside the marginalized disability system and empowers them to contribute to society rather than to only receive services.

Richard Gehring is the president of the Buffalo and Erie County Meals on Wheels organization. The slogan on his business card, *Touching Lives with Food and Friendship,* suggests that this is a philosophy that goes well beyond just supplying people with nutrition. It reflects a fundamental human need to take care of one another, and no one should be excluded from that opportunity to give. Gehring notes:

All home-delivered meal programs in the United States provide food for the body and soul and are often the only connection the recipient has with the outside world. We all touch lives with food and friendship one meal at a time. These phrases show up in all our materials: "Delivering food and friendship, "touching lives with food and friendship," "love in action," "dispensing calories as well as concern," "the visit is often more important than the meal." Those aren't just slogans; they are our philosophy.

As the song suggests, people often want to go where everybody knows their name, someplace where people look up with a smile when they walk through the door. Think of going home and hearing your mother say, "I'm making your favorite." How about walking into your local café haunt to have the server acknowledge you with the question, "Will you have your usual?" That sense of belonging wraps around you and warms you up like a bowl of hot soup. At that moment, you feel like you are the most important person in the room. Whether you are the one offering or the one receiving, being on either end is a gift of hospitality and a treasured experience. It is said that "it's the thought that counts" in any sort of gift. Taking time to know and understand who will receive it may require a precious investment of attention to details such as the receiver's ethnic and cultural background, religion, and dietary preferences.

Growing Relationships

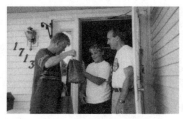

13-year-old Dayne and his dad Ron accept a bag of freshly picked tomatoes from David, whose Minnesota garden offers up a bounty for the neighborhood each fall.

This past summer, the people and staff at the home where I work in Minnesota participated in a community garden project sponsored in our town. To participate, the only prerequisites were a love of gardening and a need for a garden plot. The land, fertilizer, and water hose were furnished. All one had to do was to cultivate his plants and seeds, take care of his plot, and enjoy the produce. But to everyone's surprise, something more valued and precious than garden vegetables was cultivated and grown.

The men at our home had previous gardening experience in a horticulture therapy program when they lived at the institution. They enjoyed gardening as well as other special lunchtime meals at a local greenhouse during the summer. So we signed up for a space in the community garden. The large plot had 15 gardens in all, cared for by different people living in our town. The gardeners came from all walks of life. Some people were retired, some lived in apartments, some people had moved here from other countries, and some gardens were family projects. Each of their gardens was unique. One specialized in flowers, another had a large crop of pumpkins and gourds, and there were many with a variety of both flowers and vegetables. Going to the garden was one of the most anticipated activities each week. Our vegetables were growing beautifully, and, without even realizing it, we enjoyed meeting new people and making new friends by all sharing a common interest. Along with the fruits and vegetable, new relationships were also growing within our community. This great variety of people came together as one new group of friends. With the success of our gardens, we had an overabundance of beautiful tomatoes in the fall. So we created 10 gift bags of tomatoes and gave them to our neighbors. They were all so grateful and thankful. In the fall, we had a Community Garden Potluck at one of our local school buildings. All of the gardeners were invited, and each brought a dish to pass. We again shared garden tips and enjoyed our new connections. We all agreed to make this potluck supper an annual celebration of our harvest of vegetables and friendships. We can't wait until next year.
—Barb Handahl, United States

Sunday Dinner

My husband and I have a small group of friends who love to cook—well, one other couple who loves to cook and one single friend who loves to eat. We began a tradition of having Sunday night dinners, where we take turns hosting and trying out new recipes. The recipes can be anything, and anything they have been! From Stouffer's frozen lasagna and canned green beans to made-from-scratch Boeuf a la Bourguignon and roasted carrots. If one person can't make it we postpone, but rarely a week is missed. As a group of 20– and 30–somethings, all very busy trying to start our careers and families, this weekly meeting gives us a chance to stop and smell what's cookin'. Although we usually try new recipes and experiment with newly acquired cookware, that's really not the focus. It's a chance for all of us to have a standing date to take a break and enjoy the company of our friends. —Erin Schwier Stewart, United States

Communal Lessons

Over the years, it has become our custom every January to get together with a number of other music-related families. We go to a place we think is the centre of the universe called Totranui. There we all live in a sort of lodge where we share kitchen facilities. Everyone knows my son Kahurangi, his food habits, and his very vocal opinions. He's watched lots of other people as we share meals. Sometimes we share, and sometimes families do separate things at different times. Even if [he] has been a bit hostile about what is happening in the kitchen, he is still quite interested in watching how other people do things (eggbeaters and various kitchen gadgets intrigue him). But . . . all those people really helped me relax about what he is or isn't eating. They're very tolerant of his frequently stated opinions when he's discussing what he considers their barbaric way of eating. But they know him and they like him and that makes such an enormous difference. —Bronwyn Thurlow, New Zealand

CULTURAL CUISINE: TASTING DIVERSITY

People around the world have their own customs, languages, and dialects. A culture is made up of the beliefs, practices, rituals, and traditions of a group of people. We are enamored with others' ways of doing and ways of being. We are curious about how these ways are passed along to new generations by families through the practice of ordinary activities and special occasions. Mealtimes are prime examples.

The selection of food, its preparation, combinations, and purposes all are influenced by cultural dietary laws and traditions. Sometimes, these traditions are lost for people with disabilities who live away from their families and with others who may or may not be from the same culture or religious background. Sometimes, cultural beliefs and attitudes about the value of people with disabilities can influence the very presence of people with disabilities during mealtime. Some understanding and sensitivity about the role various foods play in someone's culture can help friends and caregivers understand the behavior of a person with a disability at mealtime.

Dr. Frances Burton is a professor of Anthropology at the University of Toronto in Canada. She teaches a course on the Anthropology of Food. She says:

Food is a cultural concept embracing both the nutritional—what nourishes the body according to biological requirements—and the symbolic meaning inherent in the meal, the diet, the choice of ingredients, and so on. This cultural or symbolic aspect is so powerful in the definition of what is edible, that offering a person the wrong food—something his or her culture or religion does not accept as proper intake—will make that person physically ill.

Burton remembers a particularly vivid example. It was the grand opening of the Roy Thomson Hall in Toronto. The International Monetary Fund was meeting there, and a feast had been prepared for the delegates who came from all over the world. Many of these people had come from developing countries, so that there was just enough money to send and house them and little left over for them to spend on food. The feast, therefore, would be an important event. At a certain moment, the dishes were unveiled and the delegates moved forward to enjoy the repast. Someone had forgotten, however, that international delegates would be coming from *all* over the world and had neglected to make appropriate dishes. Instead, there were scallops wrapped in bacon, shrimp, and other designated inedible seafood; pork dishes; and beef dishes. It was inedible to those whose religion classifies crustacean seafood as an abomination because the shrimp, lobster, or crab has eaten *traf*. [For sea creatures to be Kosher they must have fins and scales. So that leaves out shellfish and scavenger fish. All the rules of Kosher are based what was considered healthy at the time before proper food storage and refrigeration were available. Now, even though the original reasons for keeping Kosher don't exist, more observant Jews follow the ancient rules to carry on the tradition.] Clearly, a lot of the delegates could not eat this food. Pork is not Kosher. Hindus cannot eat beef; indeed, no vegetarian of any religious group could partake of most of the main courses of this meal. This sort of insensitivity is totally unwarranted, Burton says.

Contrast this disaster with Air Canada, which has a "special needs" menu that offers several different types of cuisine: vegan, ovo-vegetarian, gluten-free, vegetarian for Hindus, Kosher, Asian, Muslim; the list goes on. Burton says, "The accommodation for the multicultural background of customers is natural in the modern world."

Certain cultural imperatives should be acknowledged and respected, even if the individual is unable to articulate them. Understanding a person's heritage and societal perspectives about people with disabilities can help explain behaviors and attitudes that may be confusing to someone who is not of the same culture.

For example, in Sudanese families, requiring a family member with a disability to assist with chores of mealtime would show a lack of respect. To ask a male, let alone a male with a disability, to participate in food preparation would be unheard of.

This embarrassment or shame felt in such cultures is similar to that rooted in many other cultures in which it is believed that a child with a disability is a punishment from God. A Greek friend tells us, "I know there are local Greeks with disabilities who were born in my area, but very unfortunately, most of these individuals were sent away and institutionalized at a very young age, hidden from the Greek community." He offers a translation of a conversation he had with an older male relative on a recent visit to Greece: "These children are a reflection of a man's own worth or manhood, and [it is not] possible to allow for such visual representation of their deficiencies." In other words, many children were sent away: out of sight, out of mind.

Similarly, in many traditional East Indian families, a child or adult family member with a disability may not even be present at the table during mealtimes. Raffath Sayeed, a Canadian/East Indian doctor, lives in Canada and has a son with a disability. He says that in India, in many cases, people with disabilities are hidden from public view:

> *The child may be in the back room eating with the grandmother or being fed by a servant if the family is affluent. Sometimes very poor families have no choice because they only have a one-room home. The tradition is that it is the woman's role to serve. So she cooks, puts food on the table, and serves the child with a disability. In that case, the child is literally spoon-fed too much and doesn't learn to look after himself at mealtime. He waits for the mother, grandmother, or servant.*

Of course, in every culture—even in those in which disability is historically considered shameful—there are people with disabilities and families who believe that the community is not whole without all of its members. In North America, the culture of disability is steeped in institutionalization, and sometimes it takes many generations to change attitudes from a belief in segregation to one of belonging and equality.

Learn Cultural Rules and Respect People's Sensitivities

We are more aware of each other in our global community than we ever have been before. Presentation of food, manner of eating, choice of what goes with what, who eats first, where various individuals can eat—these and other customs have profound meaning and physical concomitants.

In many cultures, women may not eat with men; in others, children are not served with their elders. In China, it is rude to play with one's chopsticks. In North America, you lift your dish to receive food, something that would be considered incorrect in China. In North Africa, the Middle East, and India, one eats with the fingers of the right hand only; the left hand is reserved for toilet functions. Most members of these cultures believe that to touch a person's right hand with one's left is disgusting; to touch food with the left hand pollutes it. Imagine Dr. Burton's dismay

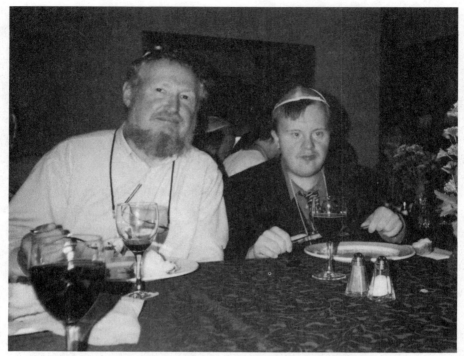

Joe and Tom enjoy a community Shabbat dinner in honor of a friend's parents' anniversary. Neither Joe or Tom is Jewish, but they chose to wear kippas in honor of Shabbat.

in Morocco when a group of villagers had invited her and her students to join them for a meal. One of the students was left-handed, and naturally used the comfortable hand without thinking. Food was served from a communal bowl. The Moroccans simply could not eat after the student had touched the food.

Never Lead with the Left

If a person has mobility difficulties or if the effects of a stroke have left the person with little or no use of the right hand, it's just "game over." The left hand is a dirty hand and it must never be used, especially to touch food. You're not to give a beggar on the street anything with your left hand, only the right. The beggar may not accept it if you present it with your left hand. —Raffath Sayeed, Canada

The people who support individuals with disabilities need to talk about respecting cultural traditions, to find out who the individual is in the context of his or her family's cultural traditions, ceremonies, and celebrations. Some effort must be made to connect with a person's family to ask about food use and meaning. Sharing of food customs provides a powerful way to include an individual in a group and to sensitize the group to another mode of operating. Many communities offer opportunities for individuals to join their ceremonies and to attend cultural food fairs. In multicultural cities and towns, there are a variety of ethnic restaurants offering not only a fun pastime but also a way to reinforce cultural identity.

Professor Burton asks her students to describe a "typical" meal. Often, her acculturated, second-generation students have to go back to a grandparent to find out how this typical meal was procured, prepared, and celebrated. The activity of doing this not only acquaints students with their individual traditions, the foods that were important, and the preparation and sharing that went into the composition of the meal but also provides classmates with a first-hand contact with a different kind of food and the cultural context in which it had meaning.

Because food is both nutritional and cultural, behaviors ancillary to the food proper have profound significance, Burton says:

> *Prayers before meals, serving honored guests, presenting special tidbits*
> *to the elderly or children, the sequence of dishes served, and the choice*
> *of complements within a meal all have a place in conveying a sense of*
> *acceptance.*

Elsewhere, she points out, in traditional cultures, the human relationship to the elements of a meal had to be respected before food could even be prepared. The Innu would thank the seal before eating any part of its body, as the seal had allowed its sacrifice to help the people.

Consider the Source

[In our culture] there are blessings for the animal that gave its life to feed everybody, much like the Native American ways. It was typical in the bush where everyone sat around the campfire to have a ceremony before you ate. The old men would talk. It was a big thing, to eat. I was brought up in a more traditional lifestyle. You appreciate the meal. I'm glad to see Murrandah is sensitive about animals. I'll cook up a kangaroo. It's pretty hard; you gotta cut it up in real thin pieces. Middle-sized ones, good eating. But the boy does kangaroo dances and won't eat kangaroo meat, so we respect that. —Goomblar Wylo, Australia

To the ancient peoples of Mexico, squash, maize, and beans (the "three sisters") were considered sacred, and together, they provided basic, nutritious sustenance. In the American Southwest, the Navajo women wore their hair in patterns recalling the stages of maturation of the squash, so that a married woman would encircle her hair over her ears as the squash blossom was at its fullest.

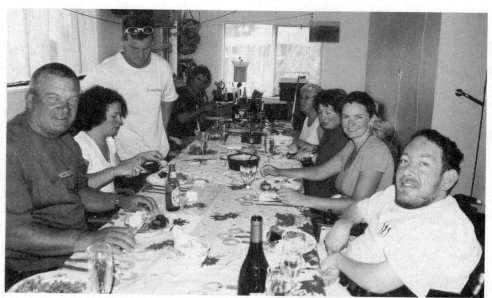

A New Zealand Christmas tea table at Te Aroha with the Pollock family is a feast that usually begins with Duncan, right, saying the Lord's Prayer in Maori.

Grandmother's Pride

The Maori in our family is on Gary's side. At special family gatherings, Gary's mom—Duncan's nanna—would ask Duncan to say grace from quite an early age. She was always very proud of Duncan and when Duncan learned to say the Lord's Prayer in Maori, she would ask him to say that as sort of a grace before the meal. She always liked to mark a family gathering by having Duncan do that for her. I think it was a chance for him to demonstrate his talents for the family, too, and she knew that.
—Kaye Pollock, Australia

What traditional dish might mean something significant to someone with a disability? A dish that speaks to them of welcome and respect can also connect them with their family and cultural community. To support someone as she marks the times of major feasts and celebratory meals in her culture and religion is a show of solidarity and respect. People are most secure when they can eat what they were raised with, which is familiar and meaningful. The smells, textures, colors, and tastes combine to create a feeling of home, of nurturance, comfort, and security. Special days can be announced in which dishes particular to an individual's childhood and culture can be made and explained to everyone, so that there is real sharing of more than just the food itself.

People come to feel a greater awareness of and appreciation for others as they become more globally in tune with traditional practices and beliefs that influence mealtimes. Learning about and helping someone celebrate his culture through food can be a rich and interesting journey for everyone involved. The one individual can feel not only accepted but also proud as the introducer of a whole new experience for everyone else.

Breaking with Tradition

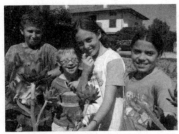

Barone brothers Luca (far left) and Andrea and their friends Claudia and Francesca inspect the produce in neighbor Luigi's artichoke patch in Pisa, Italy.

In many traditional Italian families, the parents make most decisions. It always has been that way. Then it becomes a vicious cycle; the parent makes all of the decisions, the child does not learn how to do it, and so the parent keeps doing it. If the child has a disability, then the parent wants to take care of the child even more, so it is a cultural thing. There are many families in Italy who have older children with disabilities who still live at home with Mom and Dad, who do all the laundry and cooking and so on. The child never learns to cook his own food. This is not what we want for Andrea. —Enrico Barone, Italy

A Chip Is a Chip, No Matter Where You Are

From the New Zealand Maori point of view, each *marae** would have its special food that it's known for, particularly shellfish and food from the ocean for the coastal *maraes.* Mainstream Maoridom emphasizes pork and *puha,* which is a green vegetable, a weed really, much like silverbeet. In the South Island here, the Ngi Tahu local people strongly emphasize muttonbird and oysters as a gesture of welcome for esteemed visitors. Kahurangi doesn't eat that sort of thing, but fortunately hot chips are available on nearly every corner in New Zealand! —Bronwyn Thurlow, New Zealand

*A community meeting area that includes a meeting house, dining hall, and other buildings.

Women's Work

Normally, women in my tribal community and in many others are expected to do the meal preparation. And it is a social ill for a man to be in the kitchen. The likes of me, a bachelor, will never get married within the tribe because I know how to cook. Bachelors who know how to cook are assumed to be critical troublemakers and will expect too much perfection from the women they marry just because they know the stuff! Young girls are supposed to stay away from men who spend too much time in the kitchen. This is changing, however, thank God. Otherwise, many young men like me would be in trouble! —Ben Daniel, Sudan

Exclusion: A Sign of Respect in Some Cultures

In some African cultures, excluding people with physical disabilities from performing any kind of job, including kitchen duties and housework, is supposed to be a sign of respect to the person with disabilities. African culture has socialized people with disabilities to believe that they should not do such duties. I have a friend who was a watch repairer in Southern Sudan. He used his pounds for booze. He normally earned enough to support his little sisters and brothers, an important obligation in most African cultures. But he believed that his family must clean his room, wash his clothes, and carry him home when he was intoxicated, a hobby inseparable from his habits, all because he had a disability. "Remember, I am handicap," he said to his family, "So make my food for me." Of course, there are many things he could do, but he refused, and instead, chose to exploit the values and beliefs of the society.

In more conservative cultures, parents are made to feel bad about children with disabilities. They believe that disability is a form of punishment from an African god. There is a rich set of food rituals during the three cycles: birth, marriage, and death. Well-wishers contribute cash or food. These ceremonies are not only practiced in the African black Sudanese communities in the south but also in the Arab-Sudan in the north, east, and west. Many of these cultures assume that it is rude to involve people with disabilities in any kind of activities that are demanding. —Ben Daniel, Sudan

MEALTIME AS A SUBVERSIVE ACTIVITY

Ovid once said, "Let your hook always be cast. In the pool where you least expect it, there will be fish." It takes courage, humility, and a dash of bravery for parents and family members to approach others, sometimes strangers, and invite them to be present in the life of a loved one with a disability. More than anything, it takes action. Consider this proactive family:

> A birthday party for Donna Zerr brought 35 family, friends, and well wishers to the house soon after [she had moved in from the institution.] Donna was, her mother says, "trying to squawk all the way through the party and she was hoarse for days!" Family dinners and visits are common, and there is a welcoming attitude about family members coming in to have coffee... The sense of home and belonging is something the parents rarely dared to hope for in the community. (Melberg Schwier, 1996, p. 8)

We have a friend whose daughter has profound disabilities. Her advice to other parents who want to develop connections for their children is this: Get a dog. Get a jacuzzi. Get a barbeque. Invite people over for lots of food. Whenever she took her daughter out for a walk in her chair with the family's golden retriever trotting along beside, their trips were invariably punctuated by other people out with their children and dogs. The dogs stopped and sniffed; the people stopped and sniffed (or at least the human equivalent), and contact was made. As her daughter got older, a jacuzzi was installed. Many leisurely evenings are now spent in the company of neighbors, drinks in hand, as they soak in the spa. These "carrots," dangled to entice people to come closer, are also evident in the potlucks and barbeques thrown periodically to welcome friends and neighbors. Meals shared remind people of her daughter's presence in the community, our friend says. Invitations to gather around food may prove to be a non-threatening way to include people in someone's life.

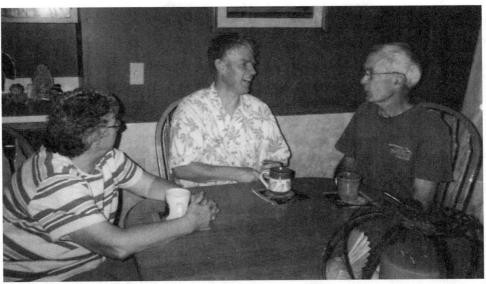

Carol and Dave are neighbors who live three blocks from David's group home in Minnesota. At least two or three times a month, they drop in for Saturday morning coffee.

If You Offer Food, They Will Come

Food was a big part of meetings with Rashaad's teachers. Got so that nothing we asked was an issue as long as they were eating! They all came for the lunches we brought in and remembered the food from meeting to meeting . . . a great way of having successful team meetings. They would all sign up, and there would be 100% attendance—even more when we sent a note around for a meeting. Then they fought for who would have the chance to teach the boys the following year. Only thing is that one has to outdo oneself from time to time. —Zuhy Sayeed, Canada

Some people hesitate to initiate connections with people who have disabilities. "If I stop in for coffee once, then it'll be an expectation that I go every day," laments one neighbor who lives beside a woman in a supported apartment living arrangement. Another family member complains, "My cousin constantly telephones to go for lunch. I'm really busy at work and I just can't drive across town to do that on a regular basis."

Once a week or once a month for lunch or coffee doesn't have to turn into a 24-hour-a-day, 7-day-a-week lifetime commitment! We tend to be afraid to hurt the feelings of someone with a disability as if they are too fragile to take the "bad news" that we can't be there all the time. Well, frankly, maybe that's not what they were asking! And maybe it hurts more to cut off all contact because we feel we can't make a full-time investment. Explain your situation, whether it is work or family commitments. Figure out something that is workable and then hold up your end of the friendship.

Occupational therapist Jitka Zgola wisely reminds us that when a little bit is given, the person has infinitely more than nothing. We know of one man with a disability who goes to the home of friends perhaps three or four times a year and once in early December for a Pizza and Christmas Tree Trimming Party, with telephone calls in between to catch up. But that's not the only social connection Francis has; in fact, years ago, his tree-trimming friends helped him to develop relationships with other people, including some at a local nonprofit organization where he now volunteers on several committees. Sometimes a significant contribution to someone's life is helping the person get connected to a variety of relationships. As they were trimming this year's tree, Francis said he might have to cut back on some of his activities because he was "getting worn out!" Do what you can and don't worry that you will be required to be all things to someone. You shouldn't try to be, because this is impossible to sustain.

Families aren't the only ones who sometimes have difficulty asking others to take part in the lives of their son and daughters. For people who were placed in institutions, attempts to reconnect with family may be tinged with sorrow and guilt. Sometimes residential staff find themselves in the delicate position of trying to orchestrate reunions. Raw memories can occasionally be soothed with mealtimes, too.

Beth Macleod is a teacher in Sydney, Australia. Her sister Margie was placed in an institution at age 5 when Beth was 2 years old. During the past few years, Beth has reconnected with her sister and admits that understanding and getting to know Margie has been a gradual process. Beth says that her head and her emotions have often been "disconnected." She was so interested in disability issues that she studied in her university classes and was inspired by a Canadian course about the need for personal networks for people with disabilities because these individuals are often isolated. The idea of calling in to see her sister whenever she attended meetings at the institution, however, just didn't occur to her:

> After I attended the course in Vancouver, the Parents and Friends Association at the institution asked me to come and give a talk about what I had learned. At that time, they used to have barbecues with the residents and family members before the meetings. I had never attended these. I arrived with my talk about how wonderful networks are and how loneliness and isolation is common in the lives of people with a disability. I arrived early, and one of the managers saw me and said, "There is someone around the back at the barbecue who would love to see you." I looked at her and wondered whom she could be talking about. It simply hadn't dawned on me to go say hello to Margie. It took that staff person to give me a kick in the right direction.

Go with the Flow

Sometimes there will be an outburst of hostility from Kahurangi, but we've learned that if you give him enough time to express his stress and work it through, he tends to handle it. I'd been on a course for a term and we were all getting together in a restaurant. He kicked up a real stink. He hated this. He hated that and the other. He wasn't going. It was a Maori ceremony so he knew there'd be lots of small speeches, song, lots of *waiata**. He wasn't going to have anything to do with it. But when he got there, he was the first one to eat. He tried three sorts of potatoes. He knows he's supposed to like kumara because he's Maori, but he doesn't. But mashed potatoes are all right. He came back with his plate piled high and I visited with people over his head while he ate. When it was my turn to receive things and sing songs about it, he was up there joining in and thoroughly enjoyed himself. —Bronwyn Thurlow, New Zealand

* Maori music

Grocery Store Contact

Sue, a staff support person in our agency, takes David and Darvin grocery shopping at Hy-Vee. She does this often. When Sue came back with David the last time, she said she invited a Hy-Vee staff lady that has become friends with David and Darvin to our Annual House Christmas Tea. She is the store hostess and helps customers to find items on their shopping list. She likes to take David or Darvin around the store with her and helps them find things. She has done this now for a while. So the Hy-Vee lady not only comes to the Tea but also she brings another friend of hers, introduces her to David and Darvin, and they all have a great time. So because Sue has taken the initiative to foster this relationship while grocery shopping and then extended an invitation to the Tea, this grocery store relationship has grown into a closer personal friendship, and David and Darvin get to know another person, too. —Barb Handahl, United States

 Make a visual shopping list. Clip pictures of items for purchase from grocery fliers or magazines. Save the labels from the food containers to use on the next shopping trip. This can also be helpful for someone with limited language or speech skills.

Coffee's On

Erin is a recent high school graduate. Loves measuring liquids. A perfectionist around the kitchen. The first dreaming/planning session with friends and families yields a connection to a small entrepreneur who runs a coffee booth in the parking lot of a garden center. Erin has beginner's luck. The Personal Network member who works at the garden center makes the introduction. Erin gets the job and her friend can keep an eye out. Erin works out back of the booth, cleaning up. Lately, she's been pouring regular coffees to ease the lineups at break. After work, she practices the art of steaming milk with her buddy from the network. Cappuccinos, anyone? (Etmanski, 2000, p. 167)

A Place On the Table

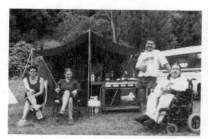

Kaye, Julie, Mike, and Duncan share New Year's Eve 1999 in Hawkes Bay, New Zealand.

When Duncan was born, they didn't close the bifida. It was sort of fashionable not to then and I think it was even an attitude of not closing surgically if the child was severely disabled because the child would likely die anyway. So Duncan's really closed over a bit on its own, but it was still quite painful to the touch. When he was 4, we decided to have the surgery and he had to lie prone, face down, for 6 weeks. We had sort of a frame with a bit of timber and padded it so he could lie on that. We'd take him everywhere in it, but when it came to mealtimes it was too low. So we just moved dishes and bowls and put Duncan and his frame right up on the table like a platter so he could be with us and see everybody! We've always been conscious of ensuring Duncan is at the same level as everyone at mealtime, so he either sat up with us in his highchair or later on a normal chair with lots of padding to prop him up. Early wheelchairs were very low and just not made for someone sitting at a dining table in mind. —Kaye Pollock, Australia

Everyone Knows Dorothy

Mum and Dad have always taken Dorothy everywhere. There's a particular restaurant in Blayney. The owner often makes a fuss over Dorothy so she really loves going there. She goes to Mass; she's well known in the church group, and the priest always makes a point of welcoming her. I don't think Mum and Dad would ever think of not taking her along to a restaurant. Mum and Dad insisted on good manners from all of us, so people really appreciate Dorothy. I think if parents don't teach their children manners and how to look after themselves with a few things as much as they can, it's really not fair to the child, is it? —Robyn Hadfield, Australia

Birthday Party Tenacity

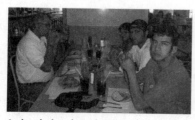

A simple lunch gathering can be a way to maintain connections.

Especially for Rashaad, we saw mealtimes as a real opportunity to get other kids to be with him. When he was young, nobody invited him for anything. He never got invited to birthday parties. We invited other people to his and then he'd never get invited back. Zuhy was getting quite disheartened, but I said don't worry, that's fine, just keep inviting them and the penny will drop sooner or later.

Then all of a sudden, the other parents said wait a minute, this is another invitation to that kid's house. And he's never been to our home? So then Rashaad started getting the calls. One guy from Lloydminster, Scott Hartnell, plays hockey in Nashville now. He told his mother, "I like hanging out with Rashaad when I come home because he knows everybody." That's why we bought Rashaad a used BMW. He can't drive, but you've got to have cool stuff around your kids with disabilities. He's never short of a driver. Same with mealtimes. Make them fun times that people like to be part of and make sure your kid is in the middle of it. —Raffath Sayeed, Canada

CHAPTER 13

BYOB

HEIDI JANZ

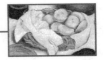

Eight years ago, when I was diagnosed with *dysphagia,* a swallowing disorder that results in particles of food being diverted from the esophagus into the trachea, potentially causing choking, in addition to my already impressive list of secondary conditions related to cerebral palsy, I knew that my life was about to change quite drastically. But amidst all the rather bewildering—not to mention alarming—talk of "silent aspiration," "laryngeal penetration," and "pooling in the vocal folds," I didn't fully realize the far-reaching impact that being suddenly restricted to eating only puréd food would have on my life.

I got my first "taste" of just how complicated my life would get when I began making arrangements for a previously-scheduled trip to Europe. I vividly remember writing a somewhat befuddled e-mail to the friend with whom I'd be staying in Cambridge. It went something like this:

> *Dear Margaret,*
> *I had a return engagement at the feeding and swallowing clinic at Glenrose on Friday. It seems that there has been some deterioration in my condition, though I'm still in very good general health (NO serious colds or lung infections all winter). However, I do seem to be having increasing difficulty getting food to go down the right way, so they've demoted me from minced food to puréed, and they suggested that I start putting thickener in my drink. They want me to EAT MY LIQUIDS AND DRINK MY SOLIDS????!!!!!*
> *(sigh) So I guess I have to ask you 2 things: 1) Do you have (access to) a food-processor/blender? 2) Am I correct in assuming that there's someplace in Cambridge where I could stock up on nutritional supplement drinks, such as Ensure?*
> *Sheesh! I must be the world's MOST DEMANDING houseguest! :-(*

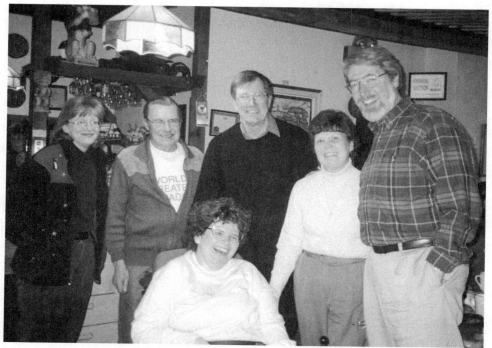

Heidi (center) meets with friends at a popular bistro.

Now, my friend, being a Most Superior TAB (Temporarily Able-Bodied person), immediately began scouring Cambridge for reasonable facsimiles of Ensure, *and* she also went out and bought a brand-new blender! Thanks to her conscientious thoughtfulness, I was able to eat very well and very safely during the time I stayed with her in Cambridge.

But the issue of eating out in restaurants—both locally and when I'm traveling—well, that can get a little more challenging. Seen from a strictly logical point of view, there seems very little reason for this to be so. After all, on a very concrete and practical level, restaurants are in the business of preparing and serving food. It would therefore stand to reason that such establishments would automatically have certain standard pieces of equipment—such as blenders and food processors—to use in food preparation. Alas, however, as is all too often the case for people living with disabilities in a TAB-centered world, reason and logic have very little bearing on the way things actually are. Consequently, I have come across some pretty illogical—and sometimes downright *bizarre*—obstacles in my ever-ongoing quest for culinary accessibility.

While the prevalence and persistence of these obstacles can, from time to time, become somewhat discouraging, the sheer outlandishness of the situations that they precipitate are often the source of great amusement—in retrospect. For example, I vividly remember a weekend trip I took to Jasper with a colleague from the university. We needed to decide where to go for dinner. But in addition to all of the *normal* accessibility questions ("Do you have a ramp?" and "Is your washroom wheelchair-accessible?"), I had to instruct my colleague to throw in the *slightly* less conventional question, "And, oh yes, do you have a blender?" At this last question, my colleague, an as-yet uninitiated TAB, would invariably have to bite her lip to keep from bursting out laughing. She said she felt like Bart Simpson making crank phone calls. After all, what sort of restaurant WOULDN'T have a blender? Well, as my colleague would soon learn, all restaurants and all blenders are definitely NOT created equal. Among the most common and most bewildering negative responses that I've received to the blender query is, "Well, yes, we do have a blender. But it's for the bar. We can't put FOOD in it!" My all-time favorite comeback to this excuse originated with my best friend who, while accompanying me to New York for a conference, replied to the most unhelpful waitress, "Well, you do have a SINK here, don't you? Can't you WASH IT OUT afterwards?" The implication being that, if they claimed not to have a sink either, we'd best rethink our choice of restaurants! A somewhat less common, but equally bewildering, negative reply that I've received is a flat-out, "No, we DON'T have a blender or a food processor. So, I'm sorry, but we simply CAN'T puré a meal for you." Such an uncategorical denial from the manager of an upscale Italian restaurant actually reduced me to nursing a milkshake for an hour and a half at what was supposed to be an annual Boxing Day brunch. Needless to say, my friends and I will not be returning to that restaurant this Boxing Day.

Thankfully though, for every blender-hoarding, puré-phobic eating establishment, I have found *at least* half a dozen restaurants that are not only *willing* but also *eager* to do all that they can to accommodate my special dietary needs. One rather incidental and incongruous, yet heartening, indication of an accessible and accommodating attitude is the practice of garnishing the indistinguishable puréd lump of what had once been an aesthetically pleasing dish of pasta, chicken, or seafood, with fresh parsley. The dysphagia automatically prevents me from safely eating the parsley, but as I instruct my dining companion to discard it, I am inevitably cheered by the thought that this is an act that millions of "gastrically normal" people perform every day.

Speaking of instructions to TAB dining companions, this seems an opportune place to reflect briefly on some basic do's and don'ts for helping people eat. Even as I contemplate constructing such a list, I become aware of the fact that, its social aspects notwithstanding, eating is, in many ways, a very personalized, individual act. Everyone has preferences regarding what, when, and how they eat. Therefore, when helping someone else eat, it's important, first of all, to get a sense of *the individual's* preferences. For example, is it easier for her to eat with a fork or a spoon? Does she prefer large mouthfuls or small mouthfuls? Does she need rest-breaks between mouthfuls? Is there a certain side or area of her mouth that she finds easier to have food on? One can discover the answers to these kinds of questions both by asking the person and by carefully observing how the person eats. Taking the time to find out the answers to these kinds of questions will make meals much more enjoyable for everyone. In my own case, I often find it helpful to remind my TAB dining companions that small mouthfuls placed in the left side of my mouth with a spoon tend to work best.

It may seem odd, but prior to being diagnosed with dysphagia and placed on a strictly puréd diet, I never really appreciated the tremendously significant role that *eating* plays in virtually every facet of my life, especially in my professional and social life. My previous oblivion to the centrality of food and eating is all the more surprising given the fact that I come from a German heritage in which virtually *all* family and/or social gatherings are centered on food! I guess, though, that because all of my life I have required someone else's physical assistance to eat, the link between food and social interaction was, to me, almost more a matter of daily necessity rather than of specific, occasional choice. Before dysphagia, the only potential barrier preventing me from participating in the social aspects of eating was the lack of a willing individual to physically put the food in my mouth. Back then, I had to deal with inaccessible locations for social/professional gatherings, but not with intrinsically *inaccessible food.* These days, as the preceding anecdotes illustrate, a blender is as indispensable to making a food-centered gathering accessible for me as are the ramps and elevators that enable structural accessibility.

This notion of a blender becoming a primary and rather unique accessibility requirement for my participation in any kind of social or professional event involving food has had a very significant and interesting impact on a number of my friends and colleagues. Many have known me since well before I was diagnosed with dysphagia "when I could still eat." Although many, if not all, of these people are intellectually aware of the fact that cerebral palsy is not a degenerative condition, they seem to have trouble resisting the emotional sense that, because I can no longer eat solid food, I must somehow be "getting worse." For example, my doctoral supervisor, whom I've known for almost 20 years, has been known to appropriate half the dish of pâté department social functions just so he's able to give me *something.* On more than one occasion, he's told me that he finds it very emotionally difficult to see me *not eating.* This kind of emotional reaction is not totally ungrounded; medical teams have told me that, over time, the buildup of food particles being aspirated into my lungs will very likely result in my eventually developing recurrent lung infections and pneumonia. Consequently, to summarily dismiss as emotional overreaction the concerns of my friends and colleagues about my apparent "deterioration" would be less than realistic. Even so, when it comes to dealing with the emotional responses of friends and colleagues, I often find myself caught in a dilemma between a strong desire to try to reassure them by minimizing their concerns, and an obvious need to be realistic about what I *can* and *can't* eat safely.

But, in the years since I was first diagnosed as having dysphagia, I've gradually learned that the simplest and most helpful way to approach the whole issue of my latest acquired "eating challenge" is very matter-of-factly and with a sense of humor. I've found that this kind of approach goes a long way toward dispelling apprehensions and putting others at ease.

These days, whenever I'm invited to a social function involving food, my first question is, "Will this be a BYOB event?" Anyone who knows me now knows that, for me, BYOB means "Bring Your Own Blender."

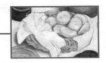

CHAPTER 14

Check the Pantry

A good cook is like a sorceress who dispenses happiness.
—Elsa Schiaparelli (as cited in Ferrer, 2004)

Teaching a person with a disability table setting skills
will give you a neat table. Teaching someone how to
be in a relationship with someone can give them a neat life.
—Dave Hingsburger

One of the goals of mealtime is to enjoy each other's company. The creation and sharing of a single dish or an entire meal is secondary. The food is the excuse, really, to be together. It provides structure and an enjoyable experience with a tangible outcome—eating the results!

In Chapter 1, Cincinnati restaurateur Larry Youse comments that a good individual dining experience has to do only partially with the taste buds. Equally important, he says, is "tasting with your eyes and ears." We think that principle should operate when people are together for mealtime, as well. Being truly present for one another means being attentive to each other's needs. It means being close enough to listen well. The Chinese character for *listening* is made up of these elements: eyes, ears, one heart, and undivided attention. This symbol should guide us as we enjoy mealtimes and each other. As we peel potatoes in the kitchen, share a plate of buffalo wings, or sit around a campfire as marshmallows wobble in the flames, we give one another the gifts of our eyes, ears, heart, and undivided attention.

Each one of us has areas in our lives in which we are less than perfect. Balancing our checkbook, exercising regularly and eating a healthy diet, changing the oil in our

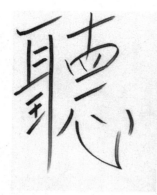

The Chinese character for listening.

car, and keeping in touch with relatives are all chores we sometimes put off, but we know they have to be done. Yet we—and hopefully the people who love and care about us—understand these little quirks are not who we are. They do not solely define us. We still want to be valued as competent human beings. We need supports here and there to move along through our daily lives. We all hope and expect to receive help with those aspects of life we have difficulty tackling, but we also expect that support to be provided with dignity and an understanding that we are so much more than the things we cannot do. We all have tasks we cannot do alone, but there are many things we don't *want* to do alone. It's simply not as much fun.

Remember back in Chapter 5, when we said there is no one recipe for being with someone with a disability? That's because everyone is unique. Find out whom you're spending time with. We call this chapter Check the Pantry because, in the experiences of family and friends we know who have disabilities, this stock-taking is too often overlooked. We heed the advice of Jamie Oliver, the passionate chef of the Food Network's *The Naked Chef, Oliver's Twist,* and the London-based documentary *Jamie's Kitchen.* He gave this tip in one of his cookbooks and, appropriately, it comes under the heading, Make Life Easy. "Before you start cooking, I can't stress enough how

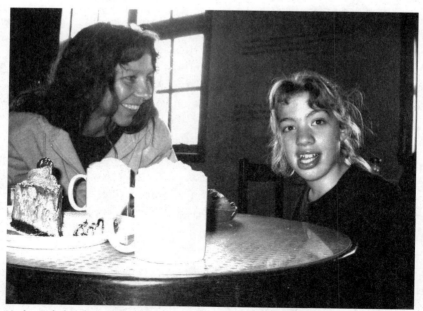

Maria and daughter Aleks stop at a Vancouver café for cake, cappuccino and hot chocolate and to enjoy life's sweetness together. Lovers of good food have something to share with whomever, whenever, and wherever.

much every kitchen should be stocked with the basics . . . [it] won't cost you the earth and will keep you in good stead. . . ." (Oliver, 2000, p. 14). Okay, we're stretching his meaning a bit, but we think this stock taking is a good rule of thumb in our relationships, too. Don't look for perfection; just know and appreciate the person as a unique individual. It doesn't cost much, and the rewards are many. Without knowing the person as a human being, without appreciating the basic ingredients, you are just going through the mechanics of human interaction. Make contact, not a checklist. Take the time to get to know this person with whom you'll spend time. Refer back to some of those questions posed in Chapter 1 as you research what makes this person tick and as you figure out ways to introduce yourself. Don't be afraid to think about what's working and not working and why as you go along. Asking "Why?" is one of the most valuable things you can do in order to better your understanding.

One young man with an intellectual disability enjoyed helping in the kitchen, particularly chopping vegetables and tearing lettuce for salads. He was precise, and all of the pieces were small and uniform. One evening, a staff member became frustrated when once again he didn't seem to understand that she wanted larger vegetable pieces for a stir-fry. Despite her efforts to show him by hand-over-hand instruction (after which she would toss the vegetables out of sight into a bowl), he kept making the pieces salad-sized. Finally, it occurred to her that a static visual cue might help. She cut a piece of each vegetable in the stir-fry size and displayed them near his cutting board. She was clear about whether she wanted him to help make a salad or stir-fry and then showed him how he could refer to the prototype. She even thought to place chopsticks near him on the counter. He then understood the difference. Sometimes, the simplest answer is sitting right in front of us, and it has little to do with a diagnosis.

 Commercial plate guards that help keep food from being pushed off can be orthopedic-looking. Consider finding dishes that have narrow rims along the inside. The design serves the same purpose without drawing attention.

MAKING ESSENTIAL CONNECTIONS

In order to feel good about ourselves, to feel productive and included, all of us need essential connections. That is, ideally we all need access to

- Information (for instance, about sexuality and relationships)
- A significant person in our lives such as a mentor
- An intimate relationship, a close friend
- A group, like a church group, a recreational organization

- A meaningful role in life
- Support people around us
- A source of joy
- A system of values
- A sense of family history
- A sense of place or a feeling of belong to a community (Regional Residential Services Society, 1998, p. 71)

For some reason that remains a mystery, human services seem determined to teach people with disabilities, who often are already isolated and lonely, skills that don't always help them form and maintain interactions and relationships with other people. Instead, we teach skills such as table setting and dish washing that are not typically carried out in the company of others. To paraphrase our friend Dave Hingsburger (1998), too often we assume somehow that quality of life must depend on quantity of skill. So we *do to* people. We create program plans and do assessments and set goals, and all the while, we keep our eyes fixed on the prize: what someone will be able to do. But human beings require engagement. Maybe the prize isn't so much what the person can do, but who the person can be. And having a little fun can't hurt either!

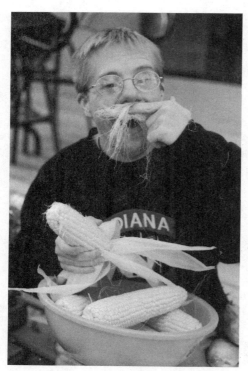

Jim cracks corn: Remember, food should be fun!

It seems to me that even though diet, physical activity, fluid intake, and sleep are all very important, there are other factors that can be almost as important and for some people maybe even more important . . . Just maybe they laugh a lot, maybe they have loving relationships, maybe they love their work and co-workers, or maybe they are just high on life. Humor and good nature can be the fuel we need for healthy emotions and can get us through many difficult and dark times in our lives. I believe some people are naturally gifted with these qualities, but I also believe that these qualities can be cultivated and nurtured if we take the time. (McPherson, 2000, p. 68)

Mealtime and all of its associated tasks can generate pride, confidence, laughter, worth, and some new talents that help to connect people with others. We've seen self-esteem rise when someone

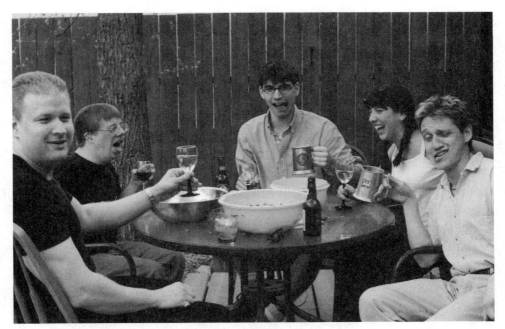

It takes true friends to appreciate a burping contest at a birthday party.

pulls their first apple pie out of the oven and proudly presents it to everyone assembled at the table. For Darlene Leister (introduced in Chapter 6), who spent 27 years in an institution, creating her first cupcake was such a source of pride; she only wished her parents were still alive to see it. The smile that a man living in a group house produces as he places a bowl of pasta he made on the table is reason enough to orchestrate the kitchen timetable and adjust the "rules of the house" to ensure that he can participate in this daily activity.

Spend time on these accomplishments—they are far more than just a cupcake or a bowl of iceberg lettuce with a few chunks of tomato and zucchini. These are true creations in every artistic sense of the word. In fact, making a dish can be a celebrated event. Something that can be done without much thought or fuss in a solitary fashion in 10 minutes by a parent or a staff member can, instead, be an occasion for togetherness—an event in itself.

Do Salad!

One great way to involve people with and without disabilities in a healthy food-making activity is to "do salad." But what do we mean by this? Here are a few suggestions to get you started and interested in salad making. Check out the produce market. Find out something new. What the heck is arugula? What do they call a zucchini in Australia? Go to a restaurant and ask a server to describe or, better yet, show

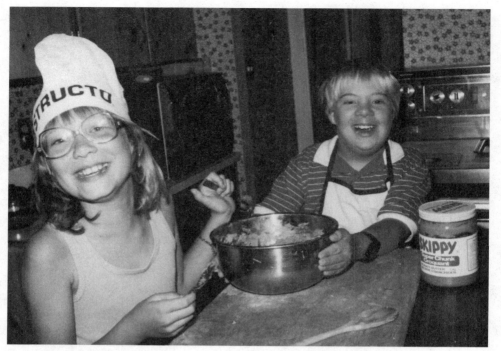

Everyone loves to bake cookies.

you how a favorite salad is made. Order the Caesar made from scratch right at your table. Try a new ethnic variety once a month. It can be a creation in the bigger cultural perspective. Try making your own dressing. Give a gift of a salad cookbook. Take photos of the preparation and the final result. E-mail them to the relatives. Make it an art form. Make it a big deal! In any case, be sure to break down the tasks so each step accomplished is an achievement.

Jim, our son/brother, has the title of Salad Maker in the family. He had an interest, we built on it, and now he takes enormous pleasure in his reputation and his place is in the kitchen, hip to hip and shoulder to shoulder with everyone else who is helping get dinner on the table. It's a portable skill, so he can pitch in and do his part for dinner in someone else's home, too.

 Tomatoes and herbs are easy to grow in a small container garden. Build the garden to meet the person's needs. Does she use a wheelchair, or would bending over to care for the plant be difficult? Maybe a raised container would allow better access.

Too much parsley in the container garden? Cut it back low on the stalk and tie up the excess bunches for drying. It's a great project to do at the kitchen table. Hang bunches in a warm, dry place. Wait about a week for them to dry completely or you can leave them hanging about the kitchen! You can do this with thyme, tarragon, sage, basil, and bay leaves, too.

Worth the Effort

Whether you are a family member who wants to get to know a relative with a disability better, a neighbor who has considered taking a "welcome to the neighborhood" cake to the young man in the basement suite next door, or a staff person responsible for supporting someone with a disability in her daily life, invest the time in learning about this person. We simply can't stress enough how important it is to make that effort.

It's okay to be uncertain. To invite yourself into someone's life is difficult. How presumptuous! What if he doesn't understand you? What if you can't understand him? What if she doesn't want to know you? How can I be friends with someone who has cerebral palsy and doesn't speak; what would we ever have in common? How would we ever go out for lunch if she takes food through a tube? What if he rejects me?

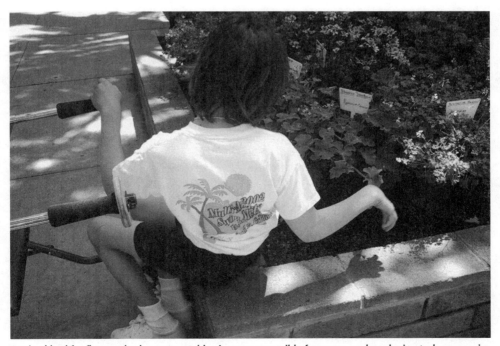

A raised bed for flowers, herbs, or vegetables is more accessible for some, and gardening tasks are easier.

As parents and family members have always known, the "ask" is hard, terrifying, in fact. Ask for what? Well, that's the beauty of mealtimes and all of its variations. They give you opportunities to ask questions about things that are almost guaranteed to interest the other person.

When you are able to put aside your qualms about being with someone with a disability and supporting that person to have a full life, including satisfying, happy mealtimes, you will be joining the community of caring individuals who truly look out for one another.

They Watch Out for You at the Bar

We see Andrea later in life . . . well, you never know what will happen. With some support, as little as possible, we would like to see him living somewhere in the community where people know him. He could go to the market to get his groceries and people will know him. We know of one young man who was fortunate because his father worked for a large supermarket, so he was able to find his son a suitable position. The son still lives with his mom, but he has a community at the supermarket. Everyone knows him, and I would like to think that even if his mom wasn't there, he would be okay because he has a community. He is very aware and good at doing things, but I noticed one day when he came off the bus that he seemed a little confused. Someone in the bar by the bus stop saw this and came out right away to help him. This is a good thing, this community where people look out for each other. They know you and they understand that you have a little problem, but it is only that you need a little help in an area, but not with everything. You still can live your life and can make your choices, but then you just need some help to make it happen.
—Enrico Barone, Italy

Think Dim Sum

As you build mealtime experiences—select menu items, venues, community opportunities, and adaptations to suit the person, the situation, and the amount of time to be shared—think dim sum. For those who've never tried this, dim sum is a Cantonese tradition of sampling an assortment of tiny morsels of different colors, fragrances, shapes, and tastes. Appropriately, the translation of dim sum means "to touch your heart."

Choose one of those, a little of that, maybe two of those. Be flexible and open. A smart cook doesn't insist on rack of lamb with garlic mashed potatoes and a fruit flan dessert if someone has an aversion to meat or the occasion is a picnic lunch in the park. Think of how mealtime works in your own home, with your own friends and family. Spur-of-the-moment occasions add variety, and the old stand-bys provide the comfort. As with dim sum, it may take many visits to determine your favorites.

If a person is resistant to eating, stop chasing the person's mouth with a spoon or pestering them with a breadstick. Give the person some space.

 Consider the person's ability or inability to switch gears if the meal consists of an item that can be eaten with the hands, such as a sandwich, and another that requires a fork, such as a side of potato salad. Serving items separately might be easier.

As you experiment with the ways you can be with someone, sharing your own memories and feelings about mealtimes that you hope that person will enjoy, remember to be open to experience the person's life, too. The joys of hospitality go both ways.

FORGING NEW FRIENDSHIPS

If you don't know a person well and she lives outside of your home, don't overlook the chance to get to know her better by accepting an invitation to have a meal in her

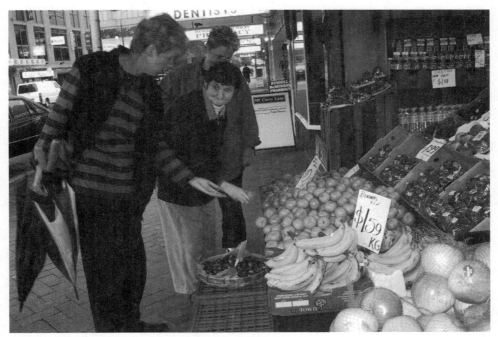

The shopping experience is part of the fun of mealtimes.

home. That might mean letting the staff at the group home or your friend's parents
or roommates know the day before to put an extra potato in the pot for you or letting
your dinner partner do that herself. By the time you come for supper, preferably
you've already introduced yourself—or have made sure the person you're connecting
with has told others about you. Remember, you're not just connecting to an individual but to the people around that person: family and perhaps other friends who care
about their happiness and security. Family and friends will want to get to know you,
to get a feel for who you are, and to feel comfortable with your relationship with their
family member or friend.

One woman who was just getting to know someone with a disability (the first
person with a disability she'd ever really tried to get to know better) said, "Cooking
and eating gave us something to do with our hands as we worked through those awkward initial steps of getting to know one another."

 If someone is distressed at mealtime, survey the environment. Are
too many choices being offered? Are the colors disturbing? Is
there an issue with the people close by? Is the food not to their
liking? Is someone staring? Is there a table leg in the way? Are you
asking the person to sit in someone else's chair? Are you truly
"with" the person, or distracted by something?

Proceed with Caution

Family and friends aren't the only people concerned about the well-being of someone
with a disability they care about. You can imagine that residential service providers
aren't keen for anybody to just walk in off the street and pull up a chair for dinner.
Some agencies are welcoming and open to family members and friends stopping in
for a visit. Others require more paperwork, especially if you're new on the scene. More
and more, police clearances or criminal background checks are being required of people who volunteer with these agencies. Nancy Wallace-Gero is the executive director
of Community Living Essex County in Essex, Ontario. People making arrangements
to have contact with someone in her agency are asked to do a number of things in addition to getting a police clearance, such as participating in an interview with a volunteer coordinator to ensure the applicant shares the same values about people with
disabilities and committing to a specific timeframe for a period of time (barring un-
foreseen circumstances). If the applicant will be driving a person in his or her vehi-
cle, the person must obtain a [report] from the [transportation department] to ensure
a good driving record. He or she might be required to provide references, as well.
Wallace-Gero notes:

> *I realize this is quite a list, but the people we support are very vulnerable
> and this is seen as a safeguard for them. Once you've been cleared, then*

our relationship with you is primarily to celebrate and thank you for what you do for people!

Given that people with disabilities can be quite vulnerable and the rate of abuse is alarmingly high, respect this and their point of view, but don't let it put you off. Use common sense and courtesy as you establish and continue your connection to the person you care about. As with any relationship, becoming a friend is a process that takes time and effort.

Step Up to the Plate; Respect All of the Rules

Dana Guernsey is the Residential Program Director with the Herkimer Area Resource Centre in Herkimer, New York. In her 21 years of experience working with people who have disabilities, she learns time and again that people are more alike than different. Making any human connection is a process, she says, that needs care and nurturing.

Understandably, residential staff members feel a great sense of responsibility for the care of people living in the agency. They can be—and should be—cautious about letting someone unknown to them through the front door. When someone interested in forming a friendship approaches them, they want to understand the motivation. Unfortunately, we still live in an era in which it is a bit unusual and even suspect for someone to seek out a relationship with someone with a disability. Guernsey notes that having worked in a residential home providing direct care early on in her career, she remembers the awkwardness between residents and staff and neighbors. She has a few suggestions that will certainly help break the ice for people who are interested in getting to know their neighbors.

- *Introduce yourself to the staff on shift and ask when you might be able to stop back to meet the house manager or supervisor.* When you meet the manager, offer information about yourself such as your name and where you live in the neighborhood. Explain what you'd like to do: Get to know the residents, or share a special interest or talent such as cooking, baking, gardening, crafts, or walking. Ask the manager what interest the residents have. Ask when would be a good time to come back to meet the residents.

- *When you meet the residents, smile, extend your hand for a handshake and be friendly.* As with anyone, first impressions are lasting, and people with disabilities can see how others are feeling even if some cannot express themselves verbally.

- *Sit and visit with folks where they're most comfortable.* Most times, residents love to share their home with visitors. Residents usually love to show off their rooms or special belongings.

- *Take time.* Be interested and listen. One to one, undivided attention is precious to anyone. Consider how much of a commitment to nurturing the friendship you are willing to make, and plan with the manager and staff when you'll visit and what activities you want to do.

- *Ask the staff's judgment about telling residents about future plans.* Some people find it hard to understand abstract concepts such as time, and that they won't see you again until "next month." Perhaps mark your next visit on the house calendar. Visual cues often work well.

- *Please don't make promises you can't keep.* Remember that staff are sometimes the only people residents know in an intimate way, and many times staff move on to other careers. Residents see many people come and go from their lives. If you truly want to form a bond with a person, remember that it hurts to be stood up or to have appointments broken without warning.

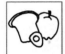 People with disabilities, especially intellectual disabilities, are plagued by the myth of the eternal child. Ask adults what they like to be called; don't assume childish versions are the preference just because other people use them. Bob shouldn't become "Bobby," Jim isn't "Jimmy," Kimberley isn't "Kimmy." And think about what to say if others insist on calling someone with a disability "honey," "sweetheart," or "sweetie." Often, strangers will do this in an effort to be friendly, but it crosses the line of intimacy.

This may seem like a long list of cautions, but it's important to remember to *relax.* Don't try to make a relationship perfect. Just be present. Let it touch your heart. Have fun! And if your experiences are positive, please share them with others. Maybe other members of your Garden Club would like to meet at a residence once in a while! Your relationship may grow to the point where you would like to have a resident visit at your house, go out for coffee or dinner, or go with you somewhere in the community. Please be patient; we're all on the same team. We want the resident to be safe and happy!

DO YOUR RESEARCH

Although most people with disabilities enjoy diets similar to yours, there are some syndromes, conditions, and disabilities that have certain metabolic characteristics. Some medications, too, influence the diets of some people. Be sure to check.

In addition, ask if there are any food restrictions because of allergies. Peanuts can be deadly to some people. Wheat, flour, and many other commonly used food items can also be dangerous. Some people are allergic to non–food items related to food production, such as latex (sometimes used in gloves for preparing food). Keep that in mind when dining out; one of the authors cannot eat food served in restaurant buffet style if the prep-cooks, chefs, or servers wear latex gloves.

If the person you are with is on a specific diet such as the ketogenic diet, do some research beforehand to determine what they can and can't eat. The ketogenic diet, for example, is high in fat, low in sugar and used to treat epilepsy; in theory, it is supposed to increase the myelination of the brain cells to decrease the "hiccups" that cause seizures.

 If someone with whom you'll be dining has strict dietary limitations because of allergies and you want to learn more about the particular allergy or allergies, go to http://www.google.com. It will take you to many supportive sites that can provide allergy-friendly recipes and restaurants.

Ask family and caregivers how they prepare meals for an individual on a ketogenic or other diet that the person likes. They will have a lot of information available and tricks for how to enjoy mealtimes together by understanding and managing restrictions. And keep in mind that special diets do not have to dampen the fun of special times. Most of us are used to celebrating special occasions with friends, family, fun, and food. These days can still be special, but they do not need to be food centered for the kids on ketogenic or other diets. For instance, at Halloween, trick-or-treat candy can be traded in for nickels to buy a new toy or rent a video. Birthday candles can be stuck into playdough and placed on a gift or the table. The rest of the family or other people dining or celebrating need not go without through the holidays; however, being sensitive to a child's unique diet therapy is warranted.

Leaving Room for More

So far, for some reason, Danny identifies birthday cake as acceptable. He likes the cupcakes I make for him. He either doesn't notice or doesn't care if he's eating something other than what other kids are eating and so far the other kids don't notice. But as he gets older, maybe it will be more of an issue, and we don't want him to feel like he's different or unusual. We might relax it a bit just to see what happens if he eats a bit of what the other kids are eating. For now, he's okay with me being in control. But at some point, he's got to learn to like pizza! What teenager doesn't like pizza? —Leigh Chou, United States

 If you are planning to dine with a person who has food texture restrictions, such as the need for a puréed-only diet or the need to have all liquids thickened because of difficulty swallowing, perhaps this is a perfect chance for you both to try those health food shakes and smoothies at juice stores.

Seeing Someone in a New Light

I really wanted to know what Margie understood. We had just finished breakfast, and I asked her if she would bring her dirty cup to the kitchen. She did this with obvious pleasure in being part of the action. Then I asked her to bring me Marion's dirty cup, and Jan's and Rachael's. As she did this, we found out for the first time that she knew all our names! Then we all started to talk about what else she could do. Marion, my other sister, said this task was easy for Margie. It wasn't even so much about what Margie could do, but it was the first time we had all started talking about her abilities and we noticed we were expecting more and wondering what else we could teach her. The nicest thing that came out of it for me was when Marion was up at the sink and Margie was really responding to her, imitating her wiping down the sink and enjoying the praise. We were all so pleased, but thought, well, there's not much opportunity to do this sort of thing at the institution where she is living, so we sort of abandoned the idea. But the next morning, we were all sitting around the table. Margie got up and went to the sink and started wiping it, looking over her shoulder with a big grin at us as if to say, look what I'm doing! She was showing off and that was something I had never seen before. It was like a whole new part of her personality that I didn't know existed. —Beth Macleod, Australia

---

 Special scrubbers with handles are available that can make it easier for someone with little hand control to wash dishes.

Treating Ourselves

We've been to Hops twice. It's sort of a steak house, and I had coupons. We've treated each other out to dinner, and we order fancy drinks and sit around and talk about the day. Laura and I went to TGI Friday's one evening, and we decided to just make it a celebration of nothing in particular. We ordered special drinks; Laura had a virgin strawberry daiquiri, and I had a virgin pina colada. We had the salad bar and just made a great evening out of it. It was fun and we made it feel like a celebration. Just because. —Rory Hoover, United States

Making Discoveries

For years when we took Ollie out, it was a serious business. We'd take him to a park for afternoon tea. There was a lot of sadness in it because of his disability and the family history. But when my partner and I got together, things changed. My partner is very playful, so she'd get Ollie laughing and play and tease him. I found out that there is a whole different way to interact with Ollie. —Stewart Howard, Australia

Discovering the Kitchen Mechanic

The whole concept of food preparation and cooking is now something Kahurangi's prepared to consider. It is a way he can be with people in the kitchen. He has a real interest in technology, so one of the most successful introductions to our family's domestic life is a butter thingy. It's like a cake ice-er, but you put the butter in and twist it around and out comes the butter. I'm not really sure what it's meant to do, other than it has, I'm sure, caused his cholesterol level to shoot straight up. He's also become competent with the bread maker, which is quite wonderful. Fortunately, he's also intrigued by the vacuum cleaner. —Bronwyn Thurlow, New Zealand

 Change positions during a task such as peeling potatoes, making salad, or even eating. For someone with limited mobility who may need support to shift positions, awareness and assistance from the person they're with is appreciated. Having pins and needles in the arms and legs isn't a fun way to finish off a meal!

Food Loosens Our Tongues

Carl can—and has—eaten two meals back to back. He was usually a quiet eater and I'm also a quiet eater, so in the beginning, our mealtime conversations were sort of, well, quiet. After a few meals together, though, we both got so comfortable with

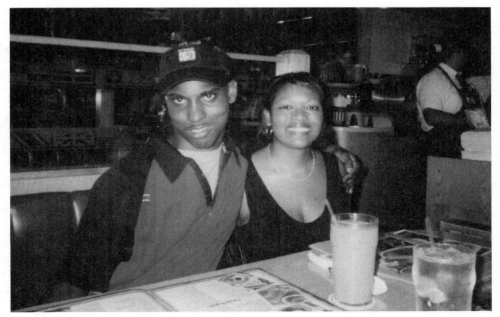

Florida buddies Carl and Aunya share good times.

each other, our conversations over a meal are now wonderful and our time together lasts longer. We laugh and listen to and understand each other, and if we don't understand each other, we have the topic of food for a good conversation during our meals. I find that most of our good talks happen over fried wonton or chicken wings or something. I've noticed that we'll even still sit there and talk after we've finished eating. I think we've let down our guard with each other. I never really thought about our outings and how they might be different, but it's true that mealtime is when maybe we totally relax and we've talked about deep things like his girlfriend, my boyfriend, and relationships and jobs and sharing and manners. All that stuff just seems to come up most naturally when we're eating. —Aunya Honore, United States

Oh, I like a lotta stuff, like Chinese buffet and chicken wings, pizza. My favorite is Kentucky Fried Chicken, and I like Burger King, McDonald's, Hometown Buffet. That's my favorite Hometown Buffet right there. They got macaroni and cheese, they got chicken wings, pizza. They got good stuff and dessert, like they got ice cream, cheesecake, I love cheesecake and Jell-O. It's all-you-can-eat sometimes but I don't eat too much. I like strawberry ice cream and hot fudge. Aunya and me, we have conversation 'bout my job, 'bout my girlfriend, things about, you know, my future life, what I want and how I'm gonna get it. She is like my nice older godsister, like that. She is a nice person. —Carl Shell, United States

 Mealtime can be a great social equalizer. If someone with a disability requires medications at mealtime, be sensitive and discreet. If dining in public or even at home, for that matter, use an attractive pillbox that could pass as a compact or glasses case. You are both diners having a nice meal, not nurse and patient.

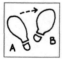 If you are taking a person with a significant disability out to eat and you don't know him well, take along a snapshot of the person in his preferred position for eating. Maybe you can jot some reminder tips on the back of the photograph that will help make the experience safe and comfortable for everyone.

If you are going out to eat, try to pick up a menu a few days before you go. You can discuss the menu items and make food choices beforehand without the distractions of the busy restaurant environment. This may eliminate some stress, if this is an issue. This also gives you and your dining partner an opportunity to discuss some of the situations that you may have to negotiate at the restaurant, and you can practice before you go.

You Just Do It

When the boy came home from the hospital, he had the tube in his nose. It came out a couple of times and I had to put it back down. It looks horrible but you just do it because you gotta do it. We could gravity feed him, but we usually just used a syringe to push the formula through down into his stomach. It took a half hour. I'd try for a half an hour every day to get him to suck, and he'd suck about 5 milliliters. One day he just took it all by the bottle. A lot of kids with the syndromes have a permanent tube into the stomach. When he was still little, we had to be careful about his palate and when he started picking up food himself to eat, I kept freaking out because I thought he'd choke. You just have to be careful. Every child's different. You just get to know what to do. —Abina Wylo, Australia

 Taking a CPR and first aid course is never a waste of time. Learn the Heimlich maneuver and other procedures to help someone who is choking.

BEST SERVED WARM

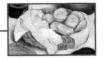

CHAPTER 15

Memorable Meals

*Ponder well on this point: The pleasant hours of our life are
all connected by a more or less tangible link, with some memory of the table.*
—CHARLES PIERRE MONSELET

Right up there with laughter, food is one of the best medicines, and some food has real healing properties. We have warm childhood memories of a favorite dish made for a special celebration, to soothe a sorrow, for a picnic or a potluck. We can close our eyes and remember what it was like when we got to lick the spoon.

Food has power. Perhaps it's because preparing and eating food is such an intimate social practice, such a sensory experience. One whiff reminiscent of Mom's German potato salad or Auntie Herma's lutefisk years later can transport us back to that occasion, that kitchen, to that person faster than Captain Picard can say "Engage."

WHAT MAKES YOU REMEMBER?

What are your memorable meals? You probably have many lodged sweetly in your mind, waiting to be conjured up by a smell or taste or bit of music that reminds you of the occasion. These are wonderful, flavorful leftovers to carry around with you. And there's always room for more! Close your eyes for a moment. Relax. Is there an occasion that comes to your mind as one so memorable that everything is bright and fresh in your mind? Here are some questions to spark memories:

- What is the occasion?

- Who is there?

- How old are you?

- What time of year is it?

- Are you inside? In the backyard? In the park? In a restaurant?

- What does it smell like?

- Are there children? Grandparents? Relatives?

- Is there music?

- What are people wearing?

- What are you wearing?

- What food do you eat?

Think about the emotions and sensations all of these memories conjure, depending on each experience: Do these memories make you feel happiness, warmth, affection, excitement, pride, anticipation? Do they give you a feeling of safety and security? Of contentment and belonging?

Think of how so many of our basic human needs are met through occasions such as these. We—as both the providers and the consumers—feed on these occasions to nurture not only our bodies but also our souls. If we examine how powerful these experiences are in our own lives—and when we begin to understand how seldom many people with disabilities have control over their experiences—we can start to understand what an influential part mealtime can play in the life of someone with a disability.

Ask your friends and family what meals or foods make them remember special times. Even if it's not a favorite, what makes a meal memorable? When your friends and family list them, ask them why those particular foods and dishes stand out above others in their minds. We'll bet most of them have an association lodged deep in their hearts from childhood that goes well beyond just the food. This is tied to times with good friends, holidays with family, and occasions when they felt safe, loved, and secure.

Because everyone's cherished memories of breaking bread and sharing meals are as unique as they are—and this is equally true for people with and without disabilities—we'd like to end this book with the voices of many people from all walks of life. When we asked some friends and family of all ages and nationalities to recall their special meals, dishes, and occasions, this is what they told us:

- Cold, raw potato wedges, lightly salted, eaten while sitting on a chair in the kitchen while Mom prepared supper. Something so simple can be passed on for generations; salted raw potatoes still taste as wonderful and the memories never diminish. It's a tradition I've passed on to my own children. —Christine, 37

- Hot milk toast, prepared only when someone had an upset stomach or the flu, had magical healing properties when Mom served it with a cool hand on the forehead. —Paula, 33

- Christmas dinner with my Polish family always included a full six- or eight-course meal, a delectable banquet of traditional Polish foods. But before anyone could take the first bite, there was the traditional passing of a large wafer of bread acquired from the church and blessed by the priest. This wafer was passed from my father at the head of the table to each one in turn in a circle around the table. As each one nibbled, he or she silently acknowledged personal forgiveness for any wrongs, any transgressions, any insults suffered at the hands of any other family member during the year. Only after each had forgiven all the others could the Christmas Feast begin. —Janet, 50

- Dad's bacon and eggs with mountains of cinnamon toast on Sunday mornings; I close my eyes and, I swear, I can smell the wonderful warm aromas. —Brian, 23

- I can't look at a can of Spam in the grocery store without vivid flashbacks of camping trips with my parents, that unmistakable smell of Spam slices frying and grease spitting over an open fire in a black cast iron skillet. The smell of spruce needles. The whine of mosquitoes. A wet tent after the rain. God, I hate Spam. —Susan, 32

- Little Joe's is a noisy, crowded Italian restaurant in San Francisco. It's in this seedy part of town and you wait in line forever. In fact, their motto is *Piogia o sole, cempré una line* (Rain or shine, there's always a line). And it's true. But you have a glass of wine while you wait. The cooks and servers are hollering in Italian, and the air is infused with aromas of garlic, tomato, pesto, and olive oil. It creates this just amazing atmosphere. The cooks are right there, throwing pasta up into the air, the flames shooting up from the burners. I framed a menu for my kitchen wall. —Bob, 29

- I spent 3 weeks in France, trying to learn the language and never being more frustrated in my life. Along with my other classmates, I visited a small village in Provence where our group was greeted by the mayor and introduced to the chef of a famous restaurant there. Half of the group went with the mayor for a tour of the town while the chef collected the rest of us and gave each of us an assignment in his kitchen. I got to peel shallots, while others cleaned mussels and prepared things I'd never seen before. It was quite the thrill to be in a professional kitchen under the watchful eye of a famous chef in France! After our hour of kitchen duty, we swapped roles with the mayor's group and had our tour of the tiny town. Later, we all dined on the meal that we had helped prepare: *moules marinere* (or mussels in white wine sauce for the non-Français). *Incroyable!* I'm convinced it was because of the shallots, but it could have been the copious amounts of wine that filled our glasses and helped make up the sauce. —Todd, 40

- Making pie dough with my grandmother. That was the best. She'd pull off a piece and sprinkle flour on the board next to her. I'd stand on a chair and roll until it was as tough as shoe leather. She sprinkled sugar and cinnamon on it and helped me cut it into stars and crescent moons. It was magic. —Kirsten, 49

- My husband and I were vegetarians (plus dairy and fish) for many years. We ate whatever was given to us by any host, but no host happened to serve steak because our friends were pretty much vegetarian, too. When we ate out, we usually ordered pasta or fish. So red meat didn't touch our lips for maybe 15 years until July of this year when we celebrated my landmark birthday. At a first-class steakhouse in the Gaslamp District of San Diego, we ordered filet mignon and a huge potato and nothing else. No salad, no sides, no dessert, no wine. After the tip, the bill came to $107.00. It was worth every cent. We savored every bite and have never enjoyed the taste of anything so much! Absence makes the buds grow fonder. We returned from that dinner as omnivores; we've eaten top-quality steak many times since but nothing to match the taste of those first precious 12 ounces. —Laura, 50

- It was late afternoon and I'd been dreaming about them all day. After patrolling several rows, I could sense I wasn't alone. Could someone be stealthily creeping along on the other side? Then, I saw them, 20 feet ahead. I quickened my pace and just as I reached for two, a hand burst through from the other side and grabbed three! I peeked over the mound and there was my brother-in-law. Artichokes were on his mind, too. He said, "You grab three more and we'll have a delicious artichoke and steak feed tonight." It was early spring in a California supermarket, and the artichokes were just coming into season. I introduced my brother-in-law Bernie to the delicious mystery of artichokes some years before as I did for my wife Gwen 25 years previous. Like so many others, they had seen artichokes but didn't know what to do with them! The artichoke is vegetable crab. When an artichoke is slowly steamed to perfection, about 20 minutes, until a fork penetrates the stump easily, it's ready. Melt some butter in a small bowl. Simply peel off one leaf at a time, dip the meaty end in butter and pull the tasty morsel off with your front teeth. When the petals are gone, take a table knife and carefully scrape off the fur around the heart, cube it, and toss the cubes in the remaining butter, then eat one at a time. Have a little red wine, a nice barbequed steak, and just savor and relish the experience. I guarantee your eyeballs will roll back in your head. —Nels, 49

- My brother and I discovered our mother had a secret hiding place for cookies. Snickerdoodles (recipe page 231). She kept them in a tin under her bed. There was nothing more thrilling than riding home on the school bus, imagining that tin waiting for us and how we could sneak a cookie or two out of it without her knowing. Arranging the ones left in the tin so she didn't notice the gap took careful concentration. —Kathy, 54

- I always loved Thanksgiving in Indiana for a lot of reasons, and I usually had the family get-together. I would get up about 2 A.M. to put on the turkey, so when we all got up in the morning, the smell of the turkey baking was wafting through the whole house. Wonderful! By mid-morning, the cooking was going full-steam ahead. One year, Dad bought a fresh turkey from a farmer who came to buy eggs at the egg plant where Dad worked. That turkey was so big I had to take off the legs and wings and take them over to Aunt Carol's to bake in her oven. Of course, the pies had been baked the day before and were in the fridge. By the time noon arrived, everybody was coming with whatever they had made to contribute to the meal. Aunt Carol usually brought baked corn and Aunt Yolande brought fresh-baked, homemade rolls. I made the cornbread dressing to stuff the turkey, but there was always one pan of oyster dressing because Grandma Farley liked it, never mind she wasn't alive anymore. I usually made Jell-O with apples, celery, and nuts in my silver-footed bowl. The table was so full of food it was hard to find room for one more dish. All the cousins were laughing and kidding around with each other. As they grew up, there was a big "thing" about the children's table. They always wanted to grow up so they could eat with the grown-ups, or at least that's what they told us. If they got together today, I'm sure there would be mention of the children's table. When the turkey was gone, nothing left but bones, the mothers cleaned up and divided up the food for everybody to take home for lunch the next day. The kids always wanted to plan for Christmas; somehow they didn't want to separate from each other. Nobody ever thought it was work; it was so much fun to be together. —Mary, 88

- My wife and I have a favorite meal. We love Kentucky Fried Chicken, but not all the coating that comes with it. We order our chicken, get two plates, and sit right there in the restaurant and pick it all off. The seasonings that seep into the chicken are wonderful, but that coating'll kill you! And we like the fact that we've pulled this off so we get what we like without clogging our arteries. —Robert, 76

- Freshly picked oranges off the tree, sliced in sections for morning breakfast. Very thin whole-grain toast with pear and ginger jam. My first breakfast after I arrived in New Zealand when I was 19. And it was the first time I had oranges straight off the tree. —Amy, 30

- Grandma Hilda and Herman had the smallest house in the city. They had a tiny metal kitchen table that sat under a small window facing the street, and the sill was lined with ceramic Red Rose Tea collectable creatures. When I was about 5 or so, Herman and I made our ritual trips to go to the confectionary (or the "Chinaman's" as he would say) to pick up some fresh French bread and cold cuts for lunch, and always Neapolitan ice cream for after. To this day I can't eat Neapolitan ice cream without thinking of them. I was always allowed to fill up a little brown paper bag with as many 1-cent candies as I wanted. The blue whales and the marshmallow strawberries burned my throat. And the pink Elephant popcorn with the prize in the box. I can still smell it if I close my eyes. Herman and I would walk home hand in hand in silence as he jingled his spare change in his pocket. By the time we got home, Grandma had made a pot of chicken noodle soup with her hand-made noodles. She just dropped her dough straight into the pot of boiling soup and made the best noodle/dumplings ever. The three of us would sit by the window and eat soup, cold cuts, and French bread smeared with way too much margarine. The bread was so chewy good, it was hard to tear apart with my teeth. Grandma Hilda and Herman chattered away in German while I sat enjoying my food, sorting through my bag of penny candies.—Samantha, 34

- Growing up in an Italian family in Toronto, I don't remember one particular memorable meal above any others. However, I do remember Sundays. I would wake up to the smell of both the freshly made espresso and the tomato sauce simmering on the stove for Sunday lunch. There was always tomato sauce in my mother's house. That smell marked the beginning of a long, leisurely day. My mother worked hard—and worked me hard—all during the week, but on Sundays, she left me alone. Thank God for religion! When I think of those Sundays, I get a warm feeling of well being and peace but, most importantly, the memory of a nurturing mother who loved and cared for her family. —Delia, 48

- For the first decade of my life, my parents, sister, brother, and I would all make an Easter pilgrimage to my great grandmother's house. She lived in a tiny little town in a tiny little house somewhere in the middle of the prairies, not far from the land she and her husband homesteaded in the mid-1930s. She lived alone but she had a garden that seemed as vast as the prairies themselves. Easter was a special time for my great grandmother, a devout Orthodox Ukrainian. I grew up knowing and understanding Catholic celebration, but on Easter we would lend ourselves to the magnificent ritual and ceremony of her beloved church. She would prepare the most intricate woven bread and carry it along with a basket of eggs, sausage, and such to be blessed during the service. After church, we would sit around the little kitchen table and eat and eat and eat. Everything was fresh from a farm nearby, the cream, flour, eggs, and meat. The mushroom sauce is something that I will only be able to relive through memory; mushrooms picked in the woods, cooked in cream fresh from the farm with dill grown in her garden. My dad would entertain us by cracking hardboiled eggs on our heads. Great Grandmother came across as a woman of the earth, with a straightforward minimalist lifestyle. But she represented a complex and difficult past. She witnessed Eastern Europe at the turn of the 20th century and lived a peasant life during World War I. She was torn from her family during the 1930s to immigrate to Canada during one of the most defining and harshest periods of modern history, the Great Depression. To watch one's children and husband die too soon was a way of life, a culture. In the shadow of this past, she would prepare for us the same simple, nourishing meals. This was food for living. If you are what you eat, then the food my great grandmother fed me became my soul. —Christopher, 28

We all meet and interact with people as we swirl through life. Now and then, we reach out as someone comes close enough, and more often than not we are glad we took the risk. Some of those people become lifelong friends, others become acquaintances, others swirl away again as the current takes them on to someone new. Each one is an unrepeatable gift that can have a profound influence on our lives. By breaking bread, opening our hearts, and spending time together—maybe over a grilled cheese sandwich—we can belong to one another.

Remember how your own memorable meals—those wonderful leftovers you carry around in your mind—allow you to conjure up people, places, events, and occasions. That's what we want to help friends and family members with disabilities nourish themselves with. Often, it is not the food itself that is the central element of mealtime meanings. Rather, the important thing is the binder—the connection—that holds to us so many of our most cherished memories of friends and family throughout our lives.

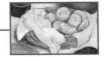

Just Desserts

Nourishment, it is clear, is a sacrament.
— VICKIE CAMMACK

We saved this story for last. It is something to savor, something to roll around in your mind as you would a nice tawny port on your tongue after a wonderful meal.

The following story by Vickie Cammack captures the essence of what food can represent between people with and without disabilities: the reason to come together, to enjoy one another's company, and to break bread for some life-giving nourishment and hospitality.

The story of Diana and Joan is far removed from the stories of feeding in institutions where boxes of false teeth were passed around for those who might need to chew and, more often, where food was simply puréed, heads were tilted back, and dinner was poured in to make it easier and faster for everyone. That sort of "mealtime" is ancient history, we hope and must believe. Today, we trust that families are involving members with disabilities in all aspects of the daily occupations of life, and that staff and volunteers in places where people with disabilities live are doing the same.

DIANA AND JOAN: THE GIFT OF COMMUNION[1]

Diana is one of the busiest people we know, on the go from dawn to dusk. She has a seat on the local school board and belongs to numerous clubs and associations. Plus she watches out for her elderly parents who live in the basement suite. To top it off, she regularly minds her own grandchildren.

---

[1]This story was excerpted from Etmanski, A. (2000). *Diana: The gift of communion* (p. 165). Vancouver, BC: PLAN; reprinted by permission.

A phone call or visit with her is likely to be interrupted by a runny nose, sticky hands, or a referee assignment. Files are scattered among the freshly baked cookies; books are balanced on the toaster. We were skeptical about her participation in Joan's network. Where would she find the time?

Still Diana insisted, attending most of Joan's network meetings, albeit on the fly. After all, she was a friend of the family.

Then there was a shift in the schedule of Joan's caregiver. She had to attend staff meetings every Friday and would be unable to assist at lunch. Replacement staff would be available on a rotating basis. Joan balked at strangers feeding her. So did her network. Diana agreed to bring lunch and to assist on an interim basis.

Four years later, Diana and Joan's lunch is the sublime interlude of their week. Diana's descriptions of the experience reminds one of the elaborate ritual associated with the Japanese tea ceremony. The lunch is prepared in the morning by Diana. She packs it carefully in a wicker picnic basket along with her antique silverware, crystal glasses and her best Limoges china, covers it with a linen cloth, and sets out for the 15-minute drive to Joan's house.

Upon her arrival, she clears the table, spreads the cloth, and sets out the dishes. In the gloomy gray days of winter, they might light candles. When the sun is out they often head out onto the deck. The table is portable; it is the tray on Joan's wheelchair. The cloth has been sewn to fit.

They look at each other; they smile. Grace. And then, with composure and mindfulness, Diana begins . . . [She helps Joan receive] spoonful after loving spoonful. Breaking bread. Being fully aware of the texture and taste. Savouring each slow and joyful bite.

"This is really for me," admits Diana. "Joan's gift allows me to close the window on my otherwise crazy week."

BIBLIOGRAPHY

Bibliography

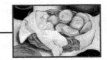

REFERENCES

American Occupational Therapy Association (AOTA). (1995). Concept paper. Service delivery in occupational therapy. *American Journal of Occupational Therapy, 49,* 1029–1031.

Bogdan, R., & Biklen, D. (1977, March/April). Handicapism. *Social Policy,* 14–19.

Bogdan, R., & Taylor, S. (1982). *Inside out: Two first-person accounts of what it means to be labeled 'mentally retarded.'* Ontario, Canada: University of Toronto Press.

Boling, E., & Smith, K. (2004). *Formative evaluation of visual instruction for individuals with intellectual disabilities: A descriptive case.* Paper presented at the meeting of the Association for Educational Communications and Technology (AECT), Chicago, IL.

Branch, S. (2004). *Autumn: From the heart of the home* (p. 42). New York: Little, Brown & Co.

Brillat-Savarin, J-A. (1970). *The physiology of taste: Meditations on transcendental gastronomy—A complete translation from the French* (p. xxxiv). New York: Liveright Publishing.

Dailey, R.H. (1983). Acute upper airway obstruction. *Emergency Medicine Clinics of North America, 1,* 261–277.

Etmanski, A. (2000). Diana: The gift of communion. In, *A good life: For you and your relative with a disability* (p. 165). Vancouver, BC: PLAN.

Ferguson, D. (1994). Is communication really the point? Some thoughts on interventions and membership. *Mental Retardation, 32*(1), 7–18.

Ferrer, L. (2004). *When food was fun, calories didn't count, candy was king, and mealtime was anytime.* New York: Artisan, a Division of Workman Publishing.

Harris, C.S., Baker, S.P., Smith, G.A., & Harris, R.M. (1984). Childhood asphyxiation by food: A national analysis and overview. *Journal of American Medical Association, 251,* 2231–2235.

Hingsburger, D. (1998). *Do? Be? Do? What to teach and how to teach people with developmental disabilities.* Eastman, PQ: Diverse City Press.

Kolpas, N. (1996). Introduction. In *Comforting foods* (p. xi). New York: MacMillan.

L'Institut Roeher Institute (1995). *Harm's way: The many faces of violence and abuse against persons with disabilities.* (p. 206). North York, ON: Author.

Lowman, D.K. (2004). Mealtime skills. In F.P. Orelove & D. Sobsey (Eds.), *Educating children with multiple disabilities: A collaborative approach* (pp. 354–356). Baltimore: Paul H. Brookes Publishing Co.

McGowan, K.G. (2002). The origins of person-centered planning. In O'Brien, J., & Lyle O'Brien, C. (Eds.) *Implementing person-centered planning: Voices of experience* (pp. 27–28, 39–40, 45–47). Toronto, Ontario: Inclusion Press.

McPherson, G. (2000). *With every breath I take: One person's extraordinary journey to a healthy life, and how you can share in it.* Edmonton, Alberta, Canada: Double M Brokerage, Ltd.

Medlen, J.E.G. (2002). *The Down syndrome nutrition handbook: A guide to promoting healthy lifestyles.* Bethesda, MD: Woodbine House.

Melberg Schwier, K. (1990). *Speakeasy: People with mental handicaps talk about their lives in institutions and in the community.* Austin, TX: PRO-ED.

Melberg Schwier, K. (1992, June/July). Then came John: The story of John McGough. *Dialect, 9.*

Melberg Schwier, K. (1994). *Couples with intellectual disabilities talk about living and loving.* Bethesda, MD: Woodbine House.

Melberg Schwier, K. (1996, September/October). It doesn't belong to the staff or parents: It's our daughters' home. *Dialect, 7.*

Melberg Schwier, K. (2000–2001,Winter). Parents focus on the joy that is our child. *Dialect, 15–16.*

Melberg Schwier, K., & Hingsburger, D. (2000). *Sexuality: Your sons and daughters with intellectual disabilities.* Baltimore: Paul H. Brookes Publishing Co.

Monselet, C.P. (2003). Our Sunday best. In R. Chronkhite (Ed.), *A return to Sunday dinner* (p. 14). Sisters, OR: Multnomah Publishers.

Oliver, J. (2000). *The naked chef takes off.* New York: Hyperion Press.

Orelove, F.P., & Sobsey, D. (1996). Mealtime skills. In F.P. Orelove & D. Sobsey (Eds.), *Educating children with multiple disabilities: A transdisciplinary approach* (3rd ed., p. 301). Baltimore: Paul H. Brookes Publishing Co.

Pavarotti, L. (1982). Some thoughts on food. In *My own story* (p. 192). New York: Warner Books.

Perske, R. (1988). *Circles of friends: People with disabilities and their friends enrich the lives of one another.* Nashville: Abingdon Press.

Perske, R. (1995). *Deadly innocence?* Nashville: Abingdon Press.

Perske, R., Clifton, A., McLean, B., & Stein, J. (1986). *Mealtimes for persons with severe handicaps* (p. 3). Baltimore: Paul H. Brookes Publishing Co.

Reid, D.H., & Parsons, M.B. (1991). Making choice a routine part of mealtimes for persons with profound mental retardation. *Behavioral Residential Treatment, 6*(4), 249–261.

Regional Residential Services Society. (1998). *Relationships and sexuality: A guide to policy for individuals with intellectual disabilities and their regional residential service providers.* Dartmouth, NS: Regional Residential Services Society and the Nova Scotia Department of Health Community Health Promotion Fund.

Roden, C. (2000). *The new book of Middle Eastern food.* New York: Knopf.

Sobsey, D., & Thuppal, M. (1996). Children with Special Health Care Needs (p. 198). *Educating children with multiple disabilities: A transdisciplinary approach* (3rd ed.). Baltimore: Paul H. Brookes Publishing Co.

Stancliffe, R.J., Dew, A., & Parmenter, T. (2002, September). *Quality service in group homes.* Unpublished address given at 13th World Congress of Inclusion International, Melbourne, Australia.

The SWIVEL Collective (2002). *Plots & pans: The book club cookbook* (pp. 133, 161). Toronto: Sumach Press.

Thuppal, M., & Sobsey, D. (2004). Children with special health care needs. In F.P. Orelove & D. Sobsey (Eds.), *Educating children with multiple disabilities: A collaborative approach* (3rd ed., pp. 354–356). Baltimore: Paul H. Brookes Publishing Co.

Vanier, J. (1989). Meals. In *Community and growth* (Rev. ed., pp. 165, 322–324). New York/ Mahwah, NJ: Paulist Press.

Whitaker, S. (1989). Point of view: Quality of life and people with a very profound handicap. *British Journal of Mental Subnormality, 35*(1), 3–7.

White, E.B. (2003). Return to the heartland. In R. Chronkhite (Ed.), *A return to Sunday dinner.* Sisters, OR: Multnomah Publishers.

Zanuck, L.F. (Producer) & Beresford, B. (Director). (1989). *Driving Miss Daisy* [Motion Picture]. United States: Warner Brothers.

Zgola, J., & Bordillon, G. (2001). *Bon appetit! The joy of dining in long-term care*. Baltimore: Health Professions Press.

RECOMMENDED RESOURCES

Readings

Butterfield, M., Arthur, M., & Sigafoos, J. (1995). *Partners in everyday communication exchanges: A guide to promoting interaction involving people with severe intellectual disabilities*. Baltimore: Paul H. Brookes Publishing Co.

Ferguson, P.M., Ferguson, D.L., & Taylor, S.J. (Eds). (1992). *Interpreting disability: A qualitative reader*. New York: Teachers College Press.

Health and Safety: Direct Care Core Competency Manual/Participant's Manual. (2001). Peachtree City, GA: McGowan Consultants.

Hingsburger, D. (1998). *Do? Be? Do? What to teach and how to teach people with developmental disabilities*. Eastman, PQ: Diverse City Press.

Hingsburger, D. (1998) *Tall tales: Self-concept and people with developmental disabilities* [audio recording]. Angus, ON: Diverse City Press. Available online from http://www.diverse-city.com.

Hingsburger, D. (2000). Panis Angelicus. *A little behind: Articles for challenge, change and catching up* (pp. 47–49). Eastman, PQ: Diverse City Press.

Laird, E. (2000). *Cooking made easy*. Boone, NC: Author.

Lowman, D.K. (2004). Mealtime skills. In F.P. Orelove, D. Sobsey, & R. Silberman (Eds.), *Educating students with multiple disabilities: A collaborative approach* (4th ed., pp. 563–608). Baltimore: Paul H. Brookes Publishing Co.

McGowan, K.G. (1998). *Solving mealtime problems*. Peachtree City, GA: McGowan Consultants.

McGowan, K.G. (2003). *Assessing persons with complex disabilities—The KMG fragility scale*. (2nd edition). Peachtree City, GA: McGowan Consultants.

Porter, B. (1998). L'Arche daybreak: An example of interfaith ministry among people with developmental disabilities. *The Journal of Pastoral Care, 52*(2), 157–165.

Relationships and sexuality: A guide to policy for individuals with intellectual disabilities and their regional residential service providers. (1998). Dartmouth, NS: Regional Residential Services Society and the Nova Scotia Department of Health Community Health Promotion Fund.

Sands, A. (2003, July). *Communion: Intimate fellowship and rapport*. Sermon delivered on July 13, 2003. Unitarian Universalist Fellowship, Harford County. Retrieved Nov. 24, 2004 from http://www.uufhc.net/s030713.html.

What's cooking? (2000). In *On my own! A resource guide for living independently* (pp. 53–66.). Toronto, ON: Canadian Abilities Foundation.

Winter, J., (1998). *Positioning for health and function*. Peachtree City, GA: McGowan Consultants.

Zgola, J., & Bordillon, G. (2001). *Bon appetit! The joy of dining in long-term care*. Baltimore: Health Professions Press.

Internet Resources

http://www.patkatz.com

Patricia Katz, of Optimus Consulting, offers a variety of resources and strategies to help people "carve out time and space for renewal" and "live a simpler life with vigor and enthusiasm."

http://www.terranova.org
Terra Nova Films has produced a teaching videotape package called *Bon Appetit! How to Create Meaningful Mealtimes in Long-Term Care,* a teaching kit consisting of two tapes and a manual for direct care staff. Contact Terra Nova Films at 9848 South Winchester Ave., Chicago, IL 60643; call 773-881-8491 or toll free: 800-779-8491; or e-mail: tnf@terranova.org.

http://www.captus.com/information/caot-webcourse-ba.htm
The Canadian Association of Occupational Therapists (CAOT) cosponsors a multimedia on-line course with Captus Press Inc. called Dining In Long-Term Care: A Primary Quality Indicator, directed to facility and program administrators, department heads, and unit directors. The program leads participants through all of the components of *Bon Appetit! How to Create Meaningful Mealtimes in Long-Term Care* (see Terre Nova films listed previously) by looking at quality care through the medium of a dining program.

http://www.bccpd.bc.ca/wdi/tips
Tips for Living Well is an on-line newsletter from the Wellness & Disability Initiative, B.C. Coalition of People with Disabilities, British Columbia, Canada. Click on Publications.

http://www.zartic.com
Go to the Zartic site and click on "Safety Guidelines" in the side menu for tips on safe steps in food handling, cooking, microwaving, and storage that are essential to avoiding food-borne illnesses.

http://www.qualitymall.org
This is an on-line "shopping mall" maintained by the Research and Training Center on Community Living, University of Minnesota, where you can find lots of free information and resources to purchase about person-centered supports for people with developmental disabilities. Each of the "Mall stores" has departments you can look through to learn about positive practices that help people with developmental disabilities live, work, and participate in our communities and improve the quality of their supports.

http://www.specialchefs.org
This site encourages people with developmental disabilities to embrace the independent living skill of food preparation to enrich their lives.

http://www.stanford.edu/group/ketodiet
Packard's Children's Hospital, Stanford University Medical Center offers this good site for information on ketogenic diets and includes a helpful FAQ section.

Miscellaneous:
You can find helpful gadgets and adaptations in a number of catalogues available on-line. The following are just a few:
http://www.theraproducts.com
http://www.enablemart.com
http://www.dynamic-living.com
http://www.abilities.ca

APPENDICES

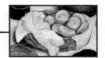

APPENDIX A

Recipes

*Cooking is like love. It should be
entered into with abandon or not at all.*
—HARRIET VAN HORNE (AS CITED IN THE SWIVEL COLLECTIVE, 2002)

All of the recipes included in this section have been selected because they're among our favorites, but we also wish to provide an array of choices for various meals and occasions. These recipes have also been chosen because they include many distinct steps that can be done in sequence or on their own as a single task to help with the overall preparation. People who have little or no experience with mealtime preparation can enjoy the sense of participation and accomplishment that small tasks—such as stirring the soup, pinching the shortening into the flour, tearing lettuce into a bowl, or loading the pickle dish—can bring.

Some recipes could pertain to more than one category. Sharing warm baking-powder biscuits in the morning with strawberry jam is equally as enjoyable as having them as a cold, easy-to-pack picnic item or with some grapes and a cup of tea in the afternoon after a shopping trip.

We present a variety of recipes, some with illustrations. These are offered with information about what equipment and utensils you will need, the ingredients, the amounts, and assembly and cooking details. You may want to use the illustrated recipes as a guide and customize others by illustrating them with your own drawings that will make sense for the person with whom you'll be working in the kitchen. At the end of Appendix A, we've provided a blank recipe template followed by three

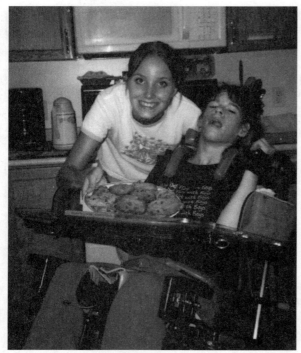

Kaitlynn, seated, and Jennifer show off a plate of freshly made cookies at Kaitlynn's house in Prince Albert, Canada.

pages of illustrations that you can trace or photocopy to tailor your own recipes if you're not a confident artist.

Individualizing recipes and cooking experiences is so important to the enjoyment of mealtimes. Joan Guthrie Medlen is a parent of a young man with Down syndrome. In her book, *The Down Syndrome Nutrition Book: A Guide to Promoting Healthy Lifestyles,* Medlen offers what we think is a great idea. As a parent, she suggests making a personal cookbook for a son or daughter with a disability. We think it would make a great accessory to mealtimes for someone of any age. Medlen writes:

Write and illustrate recipes in a method that makes sense to your child. Preparing foods is a skill of its own. It can be taught separately from literacy skills. As your child's reading skills change, so will your recipes. It makes sense not to use challenging words or multi-step directions in your recipes. Use words, symbols, and directions that are not challenging for your child as he learns to prepare foods. For now, let him focus on learning to prepare foods rather than on reading. (2002, p. 261).

A personal cookbook can be a source of pride for adults with disabilities, too. Creating such a book that is individualized and makes sense for person who will use it can be a wonderful, ongoing project. Make it a scrapbook not only of recipes but also of the memories attached to them and other mealtimes the individual has shared with family and friends. You can snap in plastic photo sleeves or envelopes and add photos, menus from favorite restaurants, or ticket stubs from events, such as the open-air Symphony in the Park when you prepared and shared that great picnic basket.

As people get together to try out new recipes and enjoy mealtimes, the favorites can be added to the cookbook. You can pencil in adaptations and make notes. Anyone who's ever had a peek at her grandmother's favorite tried-and-true recipe book knows that it's more of a filing cabinet than a book! So add your bits and pieces, too. Connections can be made with extended family to contribute; something so ordinary can be a comfortable way to reconnect. Perhaps some of the following recipes can be a starting point for the recipe book you create together. Remember, cooking may be the objective and food may be the goal, but being together and having a good time is the ultimate reward.

 Cookbooks can be awkward to handle. Buy a plate stand or book display rack at a kitchen supply store. They're cheap and you can prop open the book (including this one!) to the pages you want, for hands-free reference.

BEFORE YOU DIG IN

The main idea for including easy-to-use, illustrated recipes in this book is so that cooking together can be a supported, interactive, and interesting activity that brings people together. We do not intend for the recipes in this book to be prepared by a family member or caregiver who simply tells someone with a disability what to do next, nor are they intended to be used by someone with a disability in isolation.

Producing visual guidelines that will be completely understood by everyone is almost impossible. In fact, few if any guidelines for the creation of visual materials have been produced for individuals with disabilities (Boling & Smith, 2004). Type and level of disability varies widely as does cooking ability and experience. This is why we encourage those who will be cooking to go through a recipe they have chosen *together* and talk about it first.

What to Talk About First

Although we use a numbered sequence of tasks in each of the illustrated recipes to help guide people through the steps, notice that there are some pre-steps that should be considered initially. For example, each of the illustrated recipes features an illustrated list of ingredients and utensils to gather together first. Note that some items, whether they are food items or utensils, may not look the same where you live. In most cases something else can be used; you can discuss together what might make an acceptable substitute. You may not have a rice cooker or a wok, for instance, so some adjustments will need to be made depending what is available to you. Also note that we typically illustrate a whole food item so that it can be identified more easily; we present a drawing of a whole cabbage or a whole ginger root, for example, even though the recipe might only call for part of an ingredient. By talking about what you will need and what you have to do, you can talk about how much, what to substitute, and what you may need to buy.

Although most recipes have serving amounts (portions) suggested, you may decide to stretch it a little if someone drops in for lunch. Being together and cooking together in the kitchen isn't an exact science!

Health and Safety Issues

 Another important area to cover is health and safety. Do you have aprons to put on first? Are the potholders within easy reach? Talk about the parts of the recipe in which extra care needs to be taken, such as those that require contact with open flame, hot oil, knives, pans that have to be taken out of the oven, and so forth.

 Make sure people know how to use oven mitts. And what do you do if the smoke detector goes off? It can be quite startling and scary for someone who doesn't know what it means!

 Also talk about hygiene and staying healthy. In our house, Jim reminds us to wash our hands first in warm, soapy water so we "keep clean." We always wash hands before we begin to handle food and utensils. Talk about how to keep cutting boards clean with soapy water between cutting the chicken pieces, for example, and the vegetables for stir-fry. What happens when we have to sneeze or cough while we're preparing food?

 Wash your hands often when handling and preparing food, and before eating.

Make sure to keep raw poultry such as chicken separate from other foods. Wash cutting boards, utensils, and hands after handling raw chicken and before using those utensils again.

Making the Recipes Fit Your Needs

Depending on how familiar you both are in the kitchen, you may decide to start with recipes that are simpler than those we have included here. When you adapt your own recipes or the text recipes included in this section, use the template on pp. 251–254.

Remember to include the hand-washing illustration, the "watch out" pot holder drawing for hot pots and pans, and the "what to do when you sneeze or cough" picture. You may want to put these illustrations on a separate page that can be displayed whenever you prepare any recipe.

Abbreviations and Meanings Chart

Finally, as with most recipes, you will come across abbreviations and terms that may not be familiar to you or your cooking partner. Talk about the meaning of phrases such as *stir constantly, make a well,* and *set aside* before you get started or before you do that step. We hope you won't feel the need to memorize these, but by listing them here, you can refer to this chart if you get stuck.

Abbreviations

tsp = teaspoon	pkg = package
T = tablespoon	oz = ounce

Meanings

tin	can
make a well	make a shallow hole in the middle of your mixture
set aside	put to the side within reach for later
stir constantly	keep moving in circular motion with a spoon to keep from sticking or burning
core	cut out center with seeds in vegetables or fruit
peel	remove outer skin
fold	combine by cutting through mixture vertically and then folding sides over with flat utensil
reduce heat	turn down the flame or heat
beat	stir or whip fast
sauté	cook quickly but gently in a little hot oil stirring to prevent sticking, usually until you can see through the onions, for example
drain	pour off liquid
mince	chop into very small pieces
fry	cook in a little oil or fat in an open pan
chop	cut into small pieces
simmer	cook in liquid just below boiling point
cream	mix quickly with a spoon until soft and fluffy
dice	cut into small cubes, less than ½ inch

LIST OF RECIPES BY MEAL CATEGORY

(The recipes marked with an asterisk* appear in the illustrated section that follows each meal category)

Breakfast

Lunch

Dinner

Remember, any time you're preparing food, you must wash your hands before you start. Use soap and warm water. Turn away from food, utensils, and work areas if you have to sneeze or cough, then wash your hands again. Remember to use a potholder or oven mitt to take hot pans out of the oven.

BREAKFAST

Scrambled Eggs

Use two eggs per person.

Crack the eggs into a large bowl.

Mix thoroughly with a fork or whisk. Add salt, pepper, parsley, a few sliced mushrooms, chopped onions, chopped tomatoes, and a little shredded cheese if desired.

Spray vegetable cooking oil into large frying pan.

Turn heat up to medium-high.

Pour in egg mixture and keep stirring around with spatula, keeping the eggs from
sticking to the pan. Stir and turn constantly until eggs are firm.

Dish up on individual plates.

Some people like ketchup or hot sauce with scrambled eggs.

Servings: 1

What's in one serving?

Calories	173.55
Protein	13.92 g
Carbohydrates	2.26 g
Dietary fiber	0.29 g
Fat (total)	11.73 g
Saturated fat	3.99 g
Cholesterol	429.44 mg
Sodium	299.42 mg

Oatmeal Porridge

Instant oatmeal is really easy; just follow the directions on the packet. But real on-the-
stove oatmeal is simple, too.

1 level cup quick-rolled oats

2½ cups water

1 tsp salt

Bring water to a boil; add salt. Add oatmeal slowly, stirring constantly. Turn down
heat. Keep stirring until oatmeal is a thick paste consistency. If you like, add a
handful of raisins, currants, or cranberries to the pot while the oatmeal is cooking.
("Three-minute" oats generally take a few more minutes than what the name suggests, so don't give up too soon; the oatmeal will be watery.)

Take off heat and let stand a couple of minutes before serving

Ladle into two bowls.

Sprinkle a bit of brown sugar on top if desired. Some people like to add a little milk,
cream, or even maple syrup.

Servings: 2
What's in one serving?

Calories	153.60 g
Protein	6.40 g
Carbohydrates	26.80 g
Dietary fiber	4.24 g
Fat (total)	2.52 g
Saturated fat	0.44 g
Cholesterol	0 mg
Sodium	1173.21 mg

French Toast

1 large egg
2 egg whites
¼ cup skim milk
½ tsp vanilla extract
½ tsp ground cinnamon
⅛ tsp ground nutmeg
8 one-inch thick slices bread (French or Italian preferred, but any bread will do.)
Preheat oven to 200°.

In shallow bowl, beat egg and egg whites with whisk or fork until foamy. Add the milk, vanilla, cinnamon, and nutmeg. Beat well; set aside.

Lightly spray a large, nonstick skillet with vegetable cooking spray. Heat skillet over medium heat. Dip four of the bread slices into the egg mixture, turning to coat and draining excess mixture back into the dish.

Place bread slices in prepared pan. Cook until golden brown, about 1–2 minutes each side.

Put cooked slices on a plate. Keep in warm oven.

Dip remaining slices in egg mixture and cook as directed. Spray pan with vegetable cooking spray as needed.

Sprinkle lightly with cinnamon sugar and top with maple syrup.

Servings: 4
What's in one serving?

Calories	561.29
Protein	20.79 g
Carbohydrates	101.11 g
Dietary fiber	5.93 g
Fat (total)	7.04 g
Saturated fat	1.62 g
Cholesterol	53.31 mg
Sodium	1220.68 mg

Fried Egg Sandwich

2 slices of bread and 1 egg per sandwich.

You can either toast the bread slightly in your toaster or leave it untoasted.

Heat a small frying pan; spray with vegetable cooking oil.

Carefully crack an egg in the pan; it shouldn't snap and pop. If it does, the heat is too high, so turn it down. The white should start turning white nicely when it hits the pan.

If you don't want a runny yolk, gently poke the yolk with a fork and let it spread out while cooking.

Add salt and pepper.

When the egg looks firm, gently slide a spatula under and carefully flip it over. By cooking both sides, you avoid one side that soaks up into the bread too much.

Again, sprinkle with a little salt and pepper.

After a couple of minutes, remove with spatula and slide onto the bread. Put the other piece of bread on top and serve hot.

Some people like ketchup, hot sauce, cheese, or even barbeque sauce with their egg sandwich. This also makes a good lunch item, and is great with a bowl of soup.

Servings: 1 sandwich
What's in one serving?

Calories	221.80
Protein	10.24 g
Dietary fiber	0.53 g
Carbohydrates	23.69 g
Fat (total)	8.90 g
Saturated fat	2.42 g
Cholesterol	211.14 mg
Sodium	577.46 mg

Baking Powder Biscuits* (see pp. 206–207)

Optional: Add raisins, currants, or cranberries or some grated orange zest. For something more lunchy, how about some shredded cheese? Whole wheat flour can also be used.

Servings: 18 to 20 biscuits
What's in one serving?

Calories	81.99
Protein	1.63 g
Dietary fiber	0.34 g
Carbohydrates	10.08 g
Fat (total)	3.85 g
Saturated fat	0.80 g
Cholesterol	1.24 mg
Sodium	201.65 mg

Daphne's Homemade Muesli

1 T golden syrup

¼ cup peanut oil (or other bland oil)

½ cup brown sugar

3 cups rolled oats (slow cooking kind)

1 cup oatmeal

1 cup bran flakes

¼ cup sesame seeds

¾ cup chopped walnuts

1 cup wheat germ

1 cup cornflakes

1 cup seedless raisins (optional)

Preheat oven to 350°.

In a saucepan, gently warm golden syrup, oil, and sugar so that they mix and thin slightly.

Remove from heat. In a large, shallow roasting pan, mix rolled oats, oatmeal, bran, seeds, and nuts.

Stir in liquids, then rub in with fingertips to make an even crumb layer with no large lumps.

Place pan in oven and bake for about 15 minutes, stirring every 5 minutes. Watch carefully to avoid overbrowning. Remove from oven and cool.

Add wheat germ, cornflakes, and raisins.

Optional: Add currants, chopped dried apricots, unsalted peanuts, chopped walnuts

(This is a crunchy muesli, good served with fruit. For untoasted muesli, omit the baking step. This type is less crunchy, but good with yogurt or milk. Store in an airtight container.)

Servings: About 17 (¼ cup each)

What's in one serving?

Calories	240.54
Protein	6.39 g
Carbohydrates	34.43 g
Dietary fiber	4.26 g
Fat (total)	9.73 g
Saturated fat	1.35 g
Cholesterol	0 mg
Sodium	26.89 mg

Baking Powder Biscuits

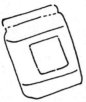   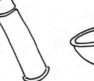

2 cups flour   3 tsp baking powder   3/4 cup milk   vegetable spray   6 T soft margarine   1 tsp salt

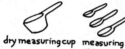

dry measuring cup   measuring spoons   liquid measuring cup

biscuit cutter   mixing spoon   pastry cutter

paring knife   sifter

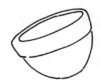

mixing bowl

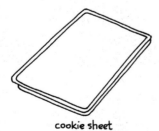

cookie sheet

1

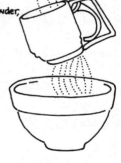

Sift the flour, baking powder, and salt together or stir it all well with a fork.

2

Cut in the margarine until it's crumbly. You can use your fingers to "pinch" the mixture until it's crumbly.

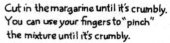

3

 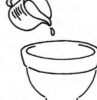

Add some of the milk; stir into flour mixture. Add the rest, making sure it is well mixed.

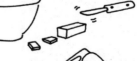 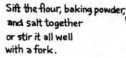

4

Place the dough on
a floured board.
Knead gently.

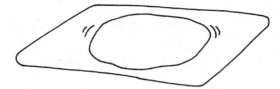

5

With a spoon or your fingers,
make "drops" or balls about
golf ball size and ...

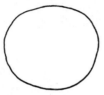

6

... drop them onto a cookie sheet
that has been lightly sprayed with
vegetable spray.

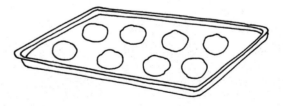

7

Bake for about 10 minutes
at 425 degrees until the
biscuits are golden brown.
Servings : 18 to 20 biscuits.

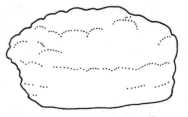

LUNCH

Grilled Cheese Sandwich

2 slices of bread per sandwich.

Put cheese slices or cut thin slices from a block of cheese in between the bread slices.

Put a frying pan on the stove and turn to low-medium heat. When it warms up, spray pan with vegetable cooking oil. Give it a good coating so the sandwich won't stick.

Put the sandwich in the pan.

In 5 minutes, lift the sandwich with a spatula, and while it is out of the pan, spray another coat into the pan.

Turn the sandwich over and put it back in the pan. The cooked side should be a golden brown.

Cook the new side for 5 minutes.

Repeat for each sandwich. Serve hot.

Optional: Our friend Todd's secret ingredient: Spread a thin layer of mustard inside the sandwich before you put the cheese on the bread.

Servings: 1 sandwich
What's in one serving?

Calories	273.97
Protein	12.34 g
Dietary fiber	0.50 g
Carbohydrates	26.10 g
Fat (total)	12.96 g
Saturated fat	7.07 g
Cholesterol	27.21 mg
Sodium	765.56 mg

Open-faced Toasted Cheese Tomato Sandwich

Make this one in the toaster oven; preheat.

1 slice of bread, 1 slice of cheese, and 1 or 2 tomato slices per sandwich. You can use sliced bread or something fancier like a baguette or specialty loaf.

Cut one thick slice for each sandwich.

Add thin slices of cheese (remember the mustard if you like it).

Slice some tomato, place one or two on top.

Sprinkle with salt and pepper.

Toast in the toaster oven for a few minutes; you can see when the cheese bubbles and starts to turn a golden brown. Don't let it go too long or the cheese will burn.

Serve hot.

Servings: 1 sandwich
What's in one serving?

Calories	140.94

Protein	6.42 g
Dietary fiber	0.59 g
Carbohydrates	14.43 g
Fat (total)	6.33 g
Saturated fat	3.55 g
Cholesterol	13.61 mg
Sodium	540.41 mg

Green Salad

This is a plain green garden salad. You can add other vegetables, but the basic recipe includes lettuce and tomatoes.

Wash a head of iceberg lettuce (the round kind) in cold water. Shake out excess water; you might even let it drain in the dish drain for a few minutes.

Cut the head of lettuce in half to make just a medium-sized salad.

Put the other half in a plastic bag and put it back in the fridge.

Tear the lettuce into small, bite-sized pieces and put in a big bowl.

Wash the tomatoes and cut off the ends with the brown bits.

Cut tomatoes in half, then half again, and keep cutting until you get bite-size chunks. Add to the bowl.

Wash and chop any of these extras: green pepper, red pepper, celery, zucchini, radishes, broccoli, cucumber. When you have added all that you want, mix it all up. When you put it on the table, don't forget to put out the salad tongs or spoons.

Servings: Several (approximately 1 cup each)

What's in one serving? (May differ depending on what vegetables are added)

Calories	20.97
Protein	1.45 g
Carbohydrates	4.18 g
Dietary fiber	1.93 g
Fat (total)	0.32 g
Saturated fat	0.05 g
Cholesterol	0 mg
Sodium	20.82 mg

Simple Greek Salad* (see page 211)

Servings: 8

What's in one serving?

Calories	103.69
Protein	4.26 g
Carbohydrates	6.85 g
Dietary fiber	1.80 g
Fat (total)	7.06 g

Saturated fat	3.18 g
Cholesterol	16.69 mg
Sodium	535.31 mg

Chickpea Salad* (see page 212)

This is a good recipe for taking along to a potluck. The recipe doubles nicely.

Servings: 6
What's in one serving?

Calories	170.06
Protein	6.49 g
Carbohydrates	28.50 g
Dietary fiber	7.11 g
Fat (total)	4.31 g
Saturated fat	0.33 g
Cholesterol	0 mg
Sodium	548.52 mg

Tri-color Pasta Salad with Vinaigrette

Cook tri-colored rotini (or other variety as you wish) pasta as per Simple Pasta directions on p. 214.

Vinaigrette: While pasta is cooking, mix up the vinaigrette. You can buy packets of pasta salad seasoning mix in the spice aisle of the grocery store.

Add seasoning to ¼ cup canola or olive oil and ½ cup white vinegar. Mix well. Note: if you don't want to make your own, a cup of Italian salad dressing will do as well.

Test pasta in about 5–10 minutes. You can try the old "throw it on the wall and when it sticks it's done" trick, or just taste it. You want it soft, but not mushy. Try for al dente (firm).

Drain pasta into a colander in the sink. Keep your face out of the steam!

Run hot water from the tap over the pasta and gently toss in the colander.

Dump into a large pasta bowl. Drizzle with oil-vinegar mixture to season. Toss thoroughly.

Optional: Add finely chopped zucchini, green and red pepper, tomato, mushrooms.

Can be served warm or chilled. Remember to mix up the leftovers well before serving again because the vinaigrette mixture tends to settle at the bottom of the bowl.

Servings: 8 (depending on quantity of vegetables, serving sizes, and dressing)
What's in one serving?

Calories	145.93
Protein	2.82 g
Carbohydrates	17.21 g
Dietary Fiber	1.07 g
Fat (total)	7.41 g
Saturated Fat	0.55 g
Cholesterol	0 mg
Sodium	2.44 mg

Simple Greek Salad

feta cheese

1/3 cup kalamata olives

oregano

pepper

salt

4 roma tomatoes

1 English cucumber

1 medium yellow onion

lemon juice

measuring cup

paring knife

spoon

fork

serving bowl

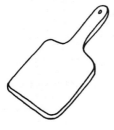
cutting board

In a serving bowl, mix up four tomatoes cut into wedges, one large cucumber cut into slices, one yellow onion cut into wedges, and 1/3 cup kalamata olives.

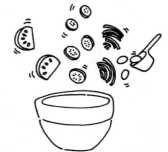

Crumble some feta cheese on top of the salad, or cut feta cheese into cubes and gently mix them in.

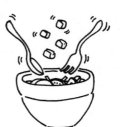

You can season the salad with a little salt and pepper, a pinch of oregano, and a squeeze of lemon juice. Serve right away.

Servings: 8

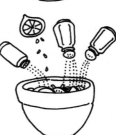

Chickpea Salad

½ tsp sugar

14 oz. can chick peas (drained)

14 oz. can black beans (drained)

14 oz. can kernel corn (drained)

1 T olive oil

¼ tsp salt & pepper

½ tsp cumin

2 T lime juice

½ cup diced red onion

¼ cup chopped Coriander/cilantro

1 ½ chopped tomatoes

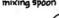
mixing spoon

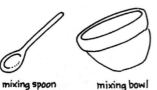
mixing bowl

mixing bowl

whisk

measuring spoons

strainer

paring knife

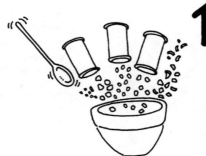

1 Put together the chickpeas, black beans, kernel corn, chopped tomatoes, diced red onion and chopped coriander/cilantro in a large bowl. Mix well.

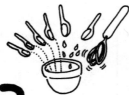

2 In a small bowl, whisk together the lime juice, olive oil, cumin, and sugar, salt and pepper.

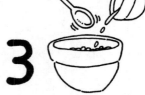

3 Pour this over the mixture and stir it until it's mixed really well. Cover it with plastic wrap or a lid and put it in the refrigerator.

DINNER

Almost All Homemade Veggie Pizza

Open and lay out the dough in 1 package of refrigerator crescent rolls in a 9-inch × 13-inch: pan. Bake as directed. Cool.

Mix together and spread on cooked crust:

1 8 oz pkg cream cheese

¼ cup low-fat mayonnaise

1 pkg ranch dressing mix

Spread ½ cup of the following finely chopped raw vegetables or whatever veggies you wish:

Broccoli, cauliflower, tomatoes, green and black olives, zucchini, cucumbers, green pepper, celery, onion, lettuce, shredded carrots.

Serve cold.

Servings: 6–8

What's in one serving? (Approximations below depend on type and quantity of vegetables per slice.)

Calories	263.43
Protein	5.59 g
Carbohydrates	17.96 g
Dietary Fiber	1.39 g
Fat (total)	18.85 g
Saturated Fat	9.74 g
Cholesterol	48.69 mg
Sodium	592.81 mg

Veggie Stir-fry and Rice

This requires chopped vegetables, just like a salad, but the pieces should be bigger.

Chop green pepper, zucchini, onion, green cabbage, pea pods, celery, carrots, broccoli, and/or cauliflower. You don't have to use all of these, but have a nice variety.

Rice: Use only a pot with a tight-fitting lid. Add 2 cups white rice (basmati is nice) to 4 cups water. Add a little salt and a tsp of vegetable oil.

Turn on the heat and bring to a boil. Stir quickly when it comes to a boil, put the lid on, turn the heat right down to simmer and don't peek! This will take about 20 minutes or so to cook.

Wash all of the veggies. Chop or slice into bite-sized chunks and small pieces. Carrots should be sliced so that they won't take too long to cook. Slice carrots and celery on an angle; they look nicer that way.

In a wok or big fry pan, add about ¼ cup olive or vegetable oil.

Turn heat to medium-high. In a couple of minutes, drop one vegetable chunk in. If it sputters, it's hot enough.

Carefully add all vegetables and keep stirring with a wooden spoon.

The heat should be high, but not so high that the vegetables will burn. Keep stirring!

Optional: You can add 1–2 tablespoons soy sauce and stir that in.

If you want to speed it up a little, turn the heat down to medium and put a lid on for a few minutes to steam the vegetables just a bit. Don't let the vegetables sit too long.

Check the rice; the water should have evaporated. If not, just put the lid back on quickly. If there's a lot of water left, turn up the heat for a few minutes.

Fluff the rice with a fork and dump into a serving bowl or onto plates. Add stir-fry veggies and serve hot. Don't forget the chopsticks!

Servings: 8

What's in one serving?

Calories	189.84
Protein	4.04 g
Carbohydrates	14.96 g
Dietary fiber	1.67 g
Fat (total)	12.65 g
Saturated fat	4.03 g
Cholesterol	15.00 mg
Sodium	498.48 mg

Hong Yan's Chinese Fried Cabbage* (see page 220)

(A Chinese friend from Chengdu province gave us this one. Caution: spicy!)

Servings: 6

What's in one serving?

Calories	73.68
Protein	2.88 g
Carbohydrates	15.02 g
Dietary fiber	4.59 g
Fat (total)	0.04 g
Saturated fat	0.01 g
Cholesterol	0 mg
Sodium	477.75 mg

Simple Pasta

Fill a medium-sized pot halfway with water.

Add 1 T vegetable oil and ½ tsp salt to the water.

Put the pot on the stove and turn the temperature on high.

Wait for the water to boil and bubble.

Put pasta noodles into boiling water. Turn down to medium heat.

Stir. Wait for the pasta noodles to get soft, but not too soft. Try for al dente (firm).

Use fork to get one or two noodles out to taste test.

When the noodles are ready, turn off the burner.

Put the colander in the sink and carefully pour the contents of the pot into the strainer.

Shake the strainer to drain all water.

Dump the pasta back into the pot and put the lid on. Put the pot back on the stove.

Serve it plain or pour some sauce from jar into pot and stir.

Serve up in bowls.

(A variety of pasta noodles can be used as well as a variety of sauces; you can buy prepared sauce or make your own: Italian, Thai, primavera. Add chopped vegetables
or chicken pieces.)

Servings: 5 (1 cup each)

What's in one serving?

Calories	192.15
Protein	5.80 g
Carbohydrates	33.88 g
Dietary fiber	1.09 g
Fat (total)	3.42 g
Saturated fat	0.56 g
Cholesterol	0 mg
Sodium	235.73 mg

Pasta e Fagiole (Pasta and Beans)* (see page 222)

(An Italian friend from Pompeii gave us this one.)

Servings: About 8 (1½ cup servings)

What's in one serving?

Calories	170.10
Protein	5.47 g
Carbohydrates	25.05 g
Dietary fiber	3.07 g
Fat (total)	5.56 g
Saturated fat	0.77 g
Cholesterol	0 mg
Sodium	23.62 mg

Skinny Fries* (see page 224)

Servings: 6 (about 6 wedges each)

What's in one serving?

Calories	211.60
Protein	3.87 g

Carbohydrates	45.63 g
Dietary fiber	3.79 g
Fat (total)	2.53 g
Saturated fat	0.36 g
Cholesterol	0 mg
Sodium	533.90 mg

Baked Chicken

There is nothing simpler than this recipe. Preheat oven to 350°.

You need a good roasting pan and a grate to put the chicken on. Spray inside the pan with vegetable oil to help with cleanup later.

Thaw a whole chicken, and then take out the neck or any stray parts the packager has put inside. Wash chicken thoroughly.

Plop into the pan, breast up.

Sprinkle on salt and pepper and some dried rosemary and put in a preheated oven at 350°. Bake for about 1½ hours, depending on size of chicken.

Advice: A good test for doneness: If it smells like baked chicken, it's probably done! Check it in about 1 hour by wiggling a leg; if it's loose and pulls away easily, it's close to being done. The chicken should reach an internal temperature of 165°.

Remember to remove skin before baking and rub the chicken with a little olive oil, or leave the skin on for flavor but remove it prior to eating the chicken since there is a lot of fat in the skin.

Servings: Approximately 4 (approximately 4 oz each)

What's in one serving?

Calories	187.11
Protein	35.18 g
Carbohydrates	0 g
Dietary Fiber	0 g
Fat (total)	4.05 g
Saturated fat	1.15 g
Cholesterol	96.39 mg
Sodium	83.92 mg

Baked Potatoes

Select the size you prefer at the farmer's market or in the produce section of the grocery store. Good bakers are the slightly long variety with deep brown, rough skins.

Scrub skins slightly and wash under the tap.

Poke each potato with a knife several times. This allows the steam to escape while it bakes. If you don't poke, or if you don't poke well enough, the potato will explode in the oven! We like baked potatoes with crispy skins, so we just put the poked potatoes straight into a 350° oven.

Time to bake varies depending on the size. Count on an hour. To test, reach in and
pinch the potato along either side. When it feels soft, it's done.

When you're ready to eat, slit the jacket down the middle to reveal all that white
fluffy inside. You can use a variety of toppings. For low-fat alternatives to butter
and sour cream, try salsa, red chili sauce, or low-fat salad dressing.

Note: Try yams or sweet potatoes; you might even be able to find something close to
the kumara that is a staple in South Pacific diets. Kumara come in yellow and pur-
ple varieties; they taste earthier than yams. We love them!

Servings: 1 potato per person

What's in one serving? (in a plain, average-sized potato)

Calories	145.08
Protein	3.06 g
Carbohydrates	33.63 g
Dietary fiber	2.34 g
Fat (total)	0.16 g
Saturated fat	0.04 g
Cholesterol	0 mg
Sodium	7.80 mg

Alanna Potatoes

(Another easy version of a baked potato that is good for barbeques.)

Peel as many potatoes as you think you need for the meal.

Tear off the same number of pieces of aluminum foil, each piece large enough to wrap
a potato.

Pour 2 T vegetable oil into a leak-proof plastic bag.

Put the potatoes in the bag, one at a time, and shake to coat with oil.

Place each potato on a piece of foil, sprinkle with salt (other seasonings if you wish),
wrap in the foil, and bake on the barbecue grill until tender (about 40 minutes for
medium-sized potatoes).

Servings: Each foil packet serves one.

What's in one serving?

Calories	227.59
Protein	3.06 g
Carbohydrates	33.63 g
Dietary fiber	2.34 g
Fat (total)	9.49 g
Saturated fat	0.70 g
Cholesterol	0 mg
Sodium	162.93 mg

Dal* (see page 226)

Good with brown basmati rice and sweet mango chutney.

Servings: 8
What's in one serving?

Calories	112.34
Protein	6.31 g
Carbohydrates	18.00 g
Dietary fiber	4.70 g
Fat (total)	2.08 g
Saturated fat	0.26 g
Cholesterol	0 mg
Sodium	305.94 mg

Fish Tacos* (see page 227)

Servings: 6
What's in one serving?

Calories	257.82
Protein	20.55 g
Carbohydrates	27.05 g
Dietary fiber	1.18 g
Fat (total)	6.86 g
Saturated fat	1.62 g
Cholesterol	26.28 mg
Sodium	420.83 mg

Skinny Man Chili* (see page 228)

Servings: 6 (about 1 cup each)
What's in one serving?

Calories	241.95
Protein	19.95 g
Carbohydrates	27.08 g
Dietary fiber	5.86 g
Fat (total)	7.47 g
Saturated fat	1.77 g
Cholesterol	59.72 mg
Sodium	1247.10 mg

Roasted Marinated Veggies

Break cauliflower, broccoli, carrots, red onions, zucchini, green pepper, and red pepper into largish pieces (2 to 2½ inches). You might also try parsnip, rutabaga, Brussels sprouts, large mushrooms, Chinese eggplant, garlic cloves, pumpkin, squash, even apples.

Drop pieces in a baggie with salad dressing. Seal bag; shake until veggies are thoroughly coated.

Place on cookie sheet sprayed with vegetable oil.

Roast at 350° for 50–60 minutes turning once at the halfway mark, until nicely browned.

Servings: 6

What's in one serving?

Calories	95.02
Protein	1.72 g
Carbohydrates	5.81 g
Dietary fiber	2.07 g
Fat (total)	7.65 g
Saturated fat	0.86 g
Cholesterol	0 mg
Sodium	356.73 mg

Hong Yan's Chinese Fried Cabbage

 rice

 1T sugar

 1T corn starch

 1/2 - 3/4 cup canola oil

 2T soy sauce

 1 1/2 - 2 T Chinese vinegar

 1 tsp salt

 green cabbage

 2 - 3 cloves garlic

 fresh ginger

 1 - 2 bunches green onions

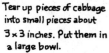 2-3 whole dried chili peppers

1 T water

---

 dry measuring cup

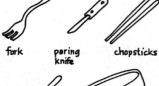 measuring spoons

liquid measuring cup

 fork

paring knife

chopsticks

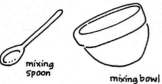 mixing spoon

mixing bowl

 rice cooker

 mixing bowl

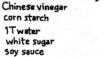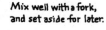 wok

1

In a small bowl, mix together:
Chinese vinegar
corn starch
1T water
white sugar
soy sauce

Mix well with a fork,
and set aside for later.

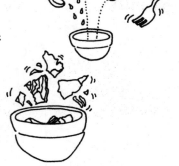

2

Tear up pieces of cabbage
into small pieces about
3 x 3 inches. Put them in
a large bowl.

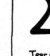

3

Peel the garlic cloves and slice them
at an angle. Peel 2-3 inches of ginger.
Slice it into little sticks, about
1 inch long. Chop 1-2 bunches of
green onion in chunks about 1 inch
to 2 inches long.
Throw away white ends.

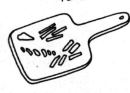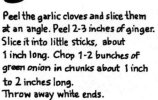

4

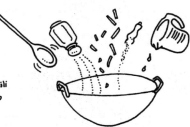

In a wok or fry pan, pour in ½ – ¾ cup canola oil.
Turn the heat on high. As the oil heats, break the dried chili
peppers into small bits with your fingers and drop them into
the oil. Add 1 tsp salt. Add the ginger and garlic.
Stir constantly and be careful of hot oil splatters.

5

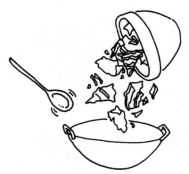

Add the cabbage and stir it all around.
Keep the heat on high and keep stirring!

Mix up the liquid
mixture with a fork.

6

Make a well in the center of the
cabbage and pour the liquid mixture in.
Stir. Cook for a few minutes.
Depending on the amount and the hardness
of the cabbage, put a lid on for a few
minutes to help soften it.

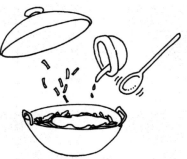

Add the green onions last.
Stir a bit more. Serve it with rice
right away when it's hot and eat.

Servings: 6
Caution: spicy!

Pasta e Fagiole (Pasta and Beans)

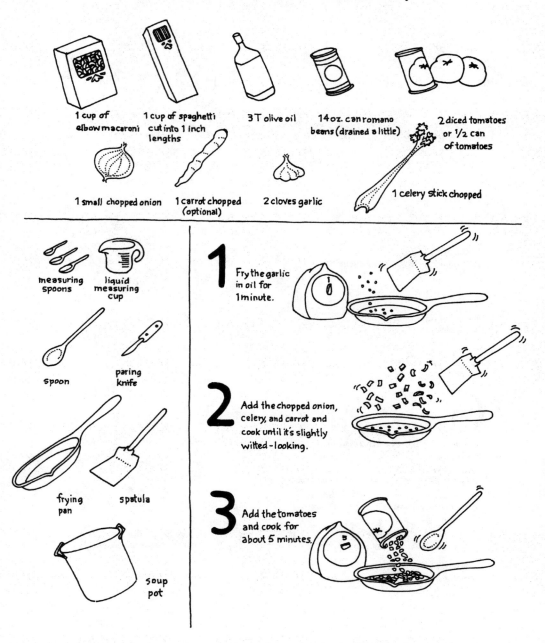

1 cup of elbow macaroni

1 cup of spaghetti cut into 1 inch lengths

3 T olive oil

14 oz. can romano beans (drained a little)

2 diced tomatoes or 1/2 can of tomatoes

1 small chopped onion

1 carrot chopped (optional)

2 cloves garlic

1 celery stick chopped

measuring spoons

liquid measuring cup

spoon

paring knife

frying pan

spatula

soup pot

1 Fry the garlic in oil for 1 minute.

2 Add the chopped onion, celery, and carrot and cook until it's slightly wilted-looking.

3 Add the tomatoes and cook for about 5 minutes.

4

Add the water and bring the mixture to a boil.

5

Add the beans and bring it back to a boil again.

6

Add the pasta and cook it all for 7 minutes or until you taste it and decide it's done!

This should come out thicker than a soup but not quite as thick as a stew. Servings: 8

To make different kinds of this soup, all you have to do is leave out the beans and change the pasta shapes. Follow the recipe up to bringing the water to a boil, then you can make different ones like these:

1) Pasta e Patate – leave out the beans and add a large cubed potato.
2) Pasta & Cauliflower – leave out the beans and add 3 cups of chopped cauliflower at the same time as the pasta.
3) Pasta & Peas – leave out the beans and add 1 cup frozen peas 2 minutes before the pasta is cooked.
4) Meatballs & Peas – leave out the pasta and beans and add precooked meatballs and peas.
5) Pasta & Chickpeas – Use chickpeas instead of beans. Add 1 cup cauliflower, 1 cubed potato, and egg noodles.

Skinny Fries

1T olive oil   1/4 tsp ground   1/8 tsp salt   ketchup or salsa   cooking spray
                black pepper

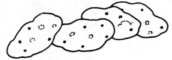

4 medium baking potatoes, cut into wedges.   2 cloves garlic, minced
Wedges can be thin or large, depending on   (optional)
what you like. Thin wedges will cook faster.

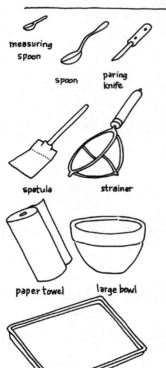

measuring spoon

spoon   paring knife

spatula   strainer

paper towel   large bowl

baking sheet

1 Put the potatoes in a large bowl. Add some cold water to cover them up so they stay crisp and don't change color. Let them sit for 15 minutes.

2 Preheat the oven to 425 F. Spray a nonstick baking sheet with cooking spray.

3 Drain the potatoes. Spread them out on a double layer of paper towels. Cover with a second layer of paper towels and press down on them with your hands to dry them.

4 Put the potatoes in a large bowl.
Sprinkle them with oil, pepper, and salt.
Toss them gently with a spoon.

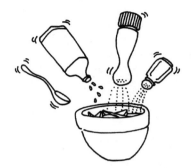

5 Lay out the seasoned potatoes
on the baking sheet.
Bake the potatoes in the oven
for 20 minutes.

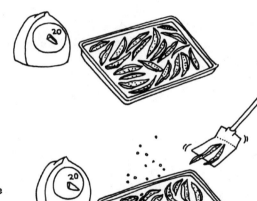

6 Use a spatula to turn potatoes over;
sprinkle on some garlic. Bake until
the potatoes are golden brown,
about 20 more minutes, turning the
baking sheet in the oven after
10 minutes for even browning.

7 Serve them hot with ketchup or salsa on the side.

Servings: 6

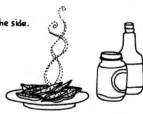

Dal

 1 cup red lentils

olive oil

 1 ½ T cumin (ground, not seed)

 mild curry paste

 salt

 2 tomatoes, chopped

 2 onions, chopped

4 cloves garlic, chopped

1 inch cube peeled fresh ginger, chopped

---

 measuring spoons

liquid measuring cup

spoons

paring knife

cutting board

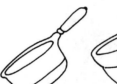 sauce pan

 mixing bowl

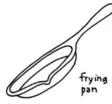 frying pan

1 Fry the onions, ginger and garlic very slowly in a little bit of olive oil.

2 When the onions are mushy, add the tomatoes. Mix together and mess it around a bit. Then add the cumin and curry paste.

3 Meanwhile, boil lentils in water. Stir quite often or they get stuck to the bottom of the pan.

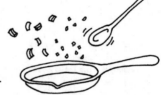

4 Mix the onion mixture and lentils together. Servings: 8, about ½ cup each.

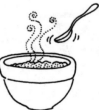

Fish Tacos

| 1½ T mayonnaise type dressing | 8 oz low fat plain yogurt | 3 oz salsa ready-to-serve | 1/16 tsp red pepper, dried, ground | 1/8 tsp black pepper, ground | 1/2 tsp cumin seed, ground | 1/2 tsp garlic powder |

 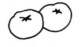

| 6 oz green cabbage, raw | 1/2 cup chopped green or red tomatoes, raw | 1 lb Atlantic/Pacific halibut fillet, raw | 6 flour tortillas | 1 T fresh lime juice & 2-3 limes |

measuring spoons | liquid measuring cup | bowl

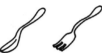

spoon | fork | paring knife

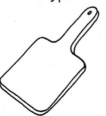

baking pan

cutting board

1 Preheat oven to 350°. Cook the fish (bake or grill) about 10-15 minutes with cumin and garlic powder sprinkled on top. When the fish looks flaky and pulls apart easily with a fork, it's done.

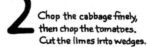

2 Chop the cabbage finely, then chop the tomatoes. Cut the limes into wedges.

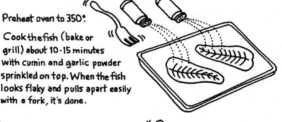

3 Make sauce:
1/2 of a small tub of plain yogurt (8 ounces)
1 1/2 T of mayonnaise
1/2 lime squeezed in (1T)
Red and black pepper to taste. Mix together.

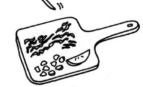

4 Warm the tortillas and put on some fish, cabbage, tomato, and sauce. Put some salsa on top. You can add black beans, rice, and lime wedges on the side.
Servings: 6

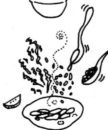

Skinny Man Chili

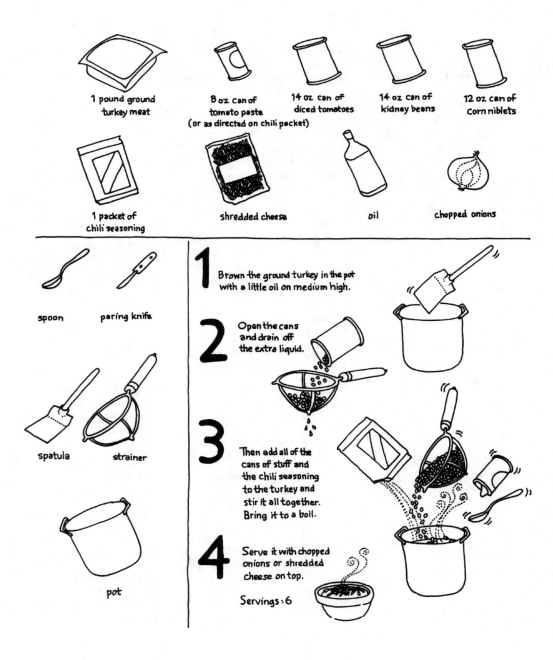

1 pound ground
turkey meat

8 oz can of
tomato paste
(or as directed on chili packet)

14 oz can of
diced tomatoes

14 oz can of
kidney beans

12 oz can of
corn niblets

1 packet of
chili seasoning

shredded cheese

oil

chopped onions

spoon

paring knife

spatula

strainer

pot

1 Brown the ground turkey in the pot with a little oil on medium high.

2 Open the cans and drain off the extra liquid.

3 Then add all of the cans of stuff and the chili seasoning to the turkey and stir it all together. Bring it to a boil.

4 Serve it with chopped onions or shredded cheese on top.

Servings : 6

DESSERTS

Smoothie

These are great for anyone and so simple to make. Use this basic recipe and just add a couple of handfuls of fruit, fresh or frozen. We like to use nonfat yogurt instead of the light cream you see called for in some recipes. Find yourself a smoothie recipe book; you can make dozens of different kinds, including veggie ones.

Basic recipe:

1 banana

3 handfuls of fruit (strawberries, melons, mangoes, blackberries, raspberries, pineapples, kiwis, diced pears, grapes, pitted cherries, you name it)

2½ cups ice (if you are using frozen fruit, ice is not necessary)

1 cup vanilla nonfat yogurt

Put the banana and fruit into the blender for about 30 seconds. Add ice and yogurt. Turn it on and off for a couple of beats to break up the ice cubes, then blend to a slushy milkshake consistency. You can also add a couple tablespoons of honey for sweetness.

Servings: 2

What's in one serving?

Calories	208.44
Protein	6.98 g
Carbohydrates	46.66 g
Dietary fiber	5.33 g
Fat (total)	0.64 g
Saturated fat	0.14 g
Cholesterol	1.83 mg
Sodium	81.92 mg

Jell-O

As the advertisements say, "There's always room for Jell-O." Make according to the simple directions on the box.

Pour powder into a bowl.

Add 1 cup boiling water. Stir.

Add 1 cup cold water. Keep stirring until thoroughly blended.

Put in the fridge, but come back and check.

Optional: When the Jell-O has started to set, sprinkle in pineapple chunks, banana slices, canned orange segments, even miniature marshmallows.

Servings: 4

What's in one serving?

Calories	80

Protein	2.00 g
Carbohydrates	19.00 g
Dietary fiber	0 g
Fat (total)	0 g
Saturated fat	0 g
Cholesterol	0 mg
Sodium	100.00 mg

Momo's Apple Dumplings

Heat oven to 350°.

Core and peel 8 small apples (about 4 oz. each)

Toss apples in bowl with ½ cup brown sugar and 1 tsp cinnamon, coating well.

Sprinkle hollow centers of apples with sugar mixture.

On lightly floured surface, roll out each biscuit from 1 package (17.3 oz.) Pillsbury Grands biscuits into 7-inch circle, using rolling pin.

Place apple in center of each circle.

Gather up dough to cover fruit. Pinch edges together to seal completely, and shape dough into apple stem and leaf, using toothpick to secure.

Place dumplings 2 inches apart on greased baking pan, and bake 30 minutes.

Remove toothpicks and let cool 5 minutes before serving.

Top with sweetened whipped cream, if desired.

Servings: 8

What's in one serving?

Calories	327.14
Protein	4.16 g
Carbohydrates	60.65 g
Dietary fiber	5.14 g
Fat (total)	8.66 g
Saturated fat	2.35 g
Cholesterol	0 mg
Sodium	610.50 mg

Fruit Salad

You can pick several of these sorts of fruits for the salad: watermelon, banana, cantaloupe, apple, honeydew melon, grapes, strawberries, blueberries, pear, orange. Try not to pick things that will just turn mushy, such as raspberries. You can scoop spoonfuls or cut into bite-sized chunks. Some things may need to be cored and peeled. Others just go in as is. Just make sure they're clean and the stems have been taken off.

Remember to make sure there is orange, orange juice, or lemon juice so that the bananas and apples don't turn brown.

Put all of the chunks and pieces into a bowl. Cover with plastic wrap and chill in the fridge until you serve. This is a nice breakfast dish, too.

Servings: About 9 (1 cup each)
What's in one serving?

Calories	70.83
Protein	0.89 g
Carbohydrates	18.01 g
Dietary fiber	2.74 g
Fat (total)	0.33 g
Saturated fat	0.05 g
Cholesterol	0 mg
Sodium	4.36 mg

Rice Krispies Squares

¼ cup margarine
5 cups marshmallows
½ tsp vanilla extract
6 cups Rice Krispies
Melt butter in large saucepan. Add marshmallows a few at a time. Stir until melted.
Remove pan from heat. Stir in vanilla. Add Rice Krispies. Mix well.
Press into pan sprayed with vegetable oil. Cool. Cut into squares.
Tip: It helps to keep your hands sprayed with vegetable cooking oil so that the mixture doesn't stick to your fingers.

Servings: About 12 (depending on the size of the squares cut)
What's in one serving?

Calories	182.02
Protein	1.21 g
Carbohydrates	34.38 g
Dietary fiber	0.06 g
Fat (total)	4.82 g
Saturated fat	0.78 g
Cholesterol	0 mg
Sodium	186.52 mg

Snickerdoodle Cookies

1 cup margarine
2 cups sugar
2 eggs
Cream margarine and sugar.
Add 1 egg at a time to the margarine and sugar.

Sift together:

2½ cups flour

2 tsp Cream of tartar

1 tsp soda

Add slowly to creamed mixture until blended. Roll into small balls the size of ping-pong balls and dip in sugar and cinnamon mixture, or drop from a spoon onto cookie sheet sprayed with vegetable oil.

Bake at 350° until golden brown.

Servings: 2 dozen

What's in one serving?

Calories	185.28
Protein	1.86 g
Carbohydrates	26.83 g
Dietary fiber	0.35 g
Fat (total)	8.06 g
Saturated fat	1.11 g
Cholesterol	15.84 mg
Sodium	159.30 mg

Duncan Pollock's Chocolate Fudge Pudding* (see pages 234–235)

Servings: 4

What's in one serving?

Calories	223.96
Protein	2.48 g
Carbohydrates	33.42 g
Dietary fiber	0.72 g
Fat (total)	9.28 g
Saturated Fat	5.70 g
Cholesterol	25.07 mg
Sodium	161.21 mg

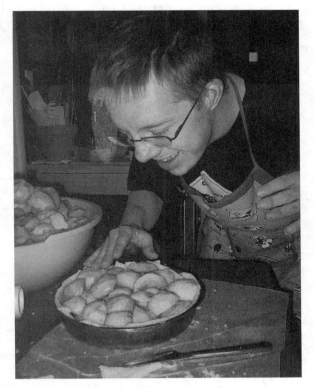

Jim concentrates on his apple pie masterpiece.

Jim's Apple Pie* (see pages 236-237)

Servings: 8

What's in one serving?

Calories	481.78
Protein	4.30 g
Carbohydrates	73.10 g
Dietary fiber	3.59 g
Fat (total)	20.42 g
Saturated fat	5.70 g
Cholesterol	17.40 mg
Sodium	140.17 mg

Duncan Pollock's Chocolate Fudge Pudding

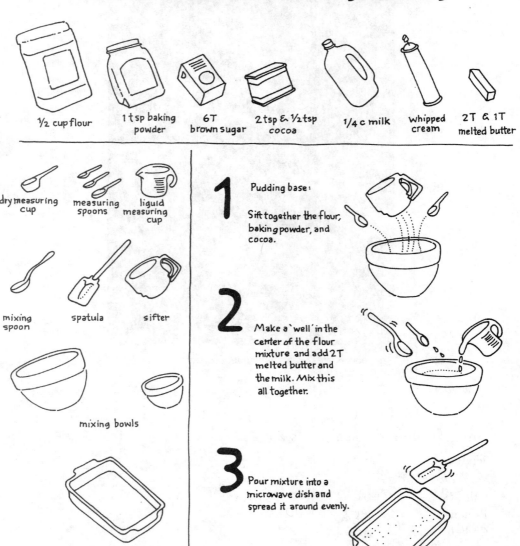

½ cup flour

1 tsp baking powder

6T brown sugar

2 tsp & ½ tsp cocoa

1/4 c milk

whipped cream

2T & 1T melted butter

dry measuring cup

measuring spoons

liquid measuring cup

mixing spoon

spatula

sifter

mixing bowls

microwave dish

1 Pudding base:

Sift together the flour, baking powder, and cocoa.

2 Make a 'well' in the center of the flour mixture and add 2T melted butter and the milk. Mix this all together.

3 Pour mixture into a microwave dish and spread it around evenly.

4 Syrup:

In a microwave bowl put:
6 T brown sugar
1 T butter
1/2 tsp cocoa
1/2 cup water

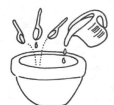

5 Put this in the
microwave for
1 minute on high.
Stir it again, then put it back in the
microwave for another minute on high.

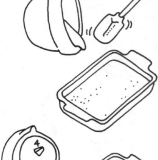

6 Then gently pour this syrup
over the pudding base.

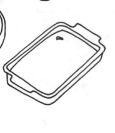

7 Cook it for 4 minutes on high,
then let it sit for 3-4 minutes.

8 Serve hot with whipped cream
or ice cream. Servings: 4

For larger batches, double the recipe,
then cook slightly elevated on a
rack on medium high for 6 minutes.

Jim's Apple Pie

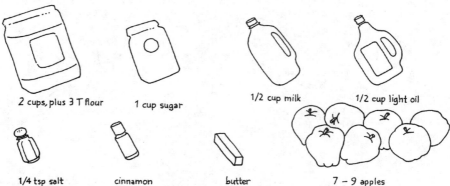

2 cups, plus 3 T flour   1 cup sugar   1/2 cup milk   1/2 cup light oil

1/4 tsp salt   cinnamon   butter   7 – 9 apples

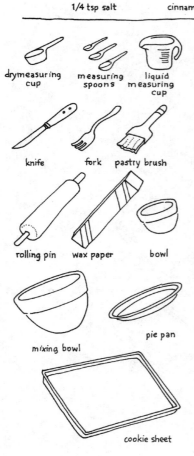

drymeasuring cup   measuring spoons   liquid measuring cup

knife   fork   pastry brush

rolling pin   wax paper   bowl

mixing bowl   pie pan

cookie sheet

1 Preheat oven to 425. Peel the apples, core, and cut into slices.

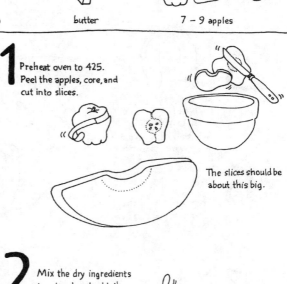

The slices should be about this big.

2 Mix the dry ingredients in a bowl and add the wet ingredients. Mix it all up with a fork. Add a little more oil if the mixture does not stick together well.

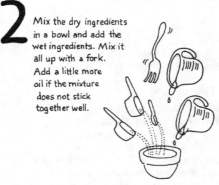

3 Form into a ball, then divide into two equal balls. Roll a crust from each ball by placing the ball between two sheets of wax paper.

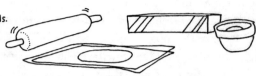

4 Place one crust in the pie pan.

5 Add the apple slices. Sprinkle cinnamon over the apples.

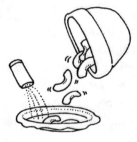

6 Place the other crust on top.
Trim and pinch the edges together.
Poke holes in the top crust.
Optional: brush melted butter on top crust.

Place pie on cookie sheet to catch any drips.

7

Bake at 425 for 15 minutes, then at 350 for 45 minutes.

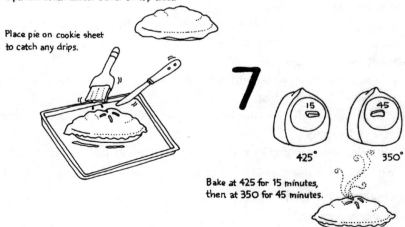

SNACKS AND NIBBLIES (APPETIZERS)

Air-Popped Popcorn

This is really easy to make in hot air machine. Measure with the cup that comes with the machine and dump the kernels carefully inside. Plug in.

Make sure bowl is positioned right and big enough to catch all of the popcorn as it flies out! Rule of thumb: ½ cup of kernels makes about 14 cups of popcorn.

Add a quick shot of vegetable spray to the hot popcorn; add salt (commercial varieties with half the sodium are available), but also experiment with other things such as cumin powder or crushed barbeque potato chips. Some people even like a sprinkling of confectioner's (icing) sugar!

Servings: 14 (about1 cup each) per ½ cup uncooked corn

What's in one serving?

Calories	30.56
Protein	0.96 g
Carbohydrates	6.23 g
Dietary fiber	1.21 g
Fat (total)	0.34 g
Saturated fat	0.05 g
Cholesterol	0 mg
Sodium	0.32 mg

Veggies & Dip

Wash a selection of vegetables: carrots, zucchini, celery, broccoli, cauliflower, green and red pepper, and/or radishes.

Cut into pieces 3"–4" in length. Cut ends off radishes and leave whole or just cut in half.

Arrange on a serving tray.

Dip: You can pour store-bought ranch dressing into a bowl. Or if you prefer to make homemade dip, try this:

Add dry contents of 1 package dry onion soup mix into 1 cup of fat-free sour cream. Mix thoroughly.

You might consider giving people their own small bowl so they can "double-dip" without offending anyone!

Servings: 16 (1 T each)

What's in one serving?

Calories	19.19
Protein	1.07 g
Carbohydrates	3.32 g
Dietary fiber	0.06 g

Fat (total)	0.04 g
Saturated fat	0.01 g
Cholesterol	1.25 mg
Sodium	65.54 mg

Celery Sticks

Wash celery ribs; cut off ends.

Cut ribs into pieces 4–5 inches in length. Shake out any excess water.

With a butter knife, fill the space in each rib, scraping off excess, with different fillings such as peanut butter, Cheez Whiz, or cream cheese sprinkled with paprika.

Arrange on a plate and serve.

Servings: 1 each

What's in one serving? (Nutritional facts change depending on the filling!)

Calories	6.40
Protein	0.30 g
Carbohydrates	6.23 g
Dietary fiber	0.68 g
Fat (total)	0.06 g
Saturated fat	0.01 g
Cholesterol	0 mg
Sodium	34.80 mg

SPECIAL HOLIDAYS AND OCCASIONS

Birthday Cake

Boxed varieties in grocery stores can be good, and the directions are easy to follow. If you'd like to try an easy, hardly ever fails chocolate scratch cake, try this one.

Doris's Devil's Food Birthday Cake

1½ cups flour
1⅓ cups white sugar
¼ tsp baking powder
¼ tsp baking soda
¾ tsp salt
½ cup cocoa
Mix these dry ingredients together in a bowl.
In another bowl, mix together:
½ cup soft margarine
¾ cup water
2 eggs
¾ tsp vanilla

Preheat oven to 350°.
Add dry ingredients a bit at a time and fold into wet mixture.
Pour cake batter into cake pan sprayed with vegetable oil. Use rubber spatula to get all of the batter out of the bowl.
Bake at 350° until toothpick inserted in center of cake comes out clean.
Let it sit on a rack to cool, and then carefully remove it from the pan and place it onto a cake serving plate.
Frost or ice as desired.
Don't forget the candles. The no-drip ones are the best.

Servings: 16 (2-ounce slices, approximately)
What's in one serving?

Calories	173.58
Protein	2.40 g
Carbohydrates	26.78 g
Dietary fiber	1.04 g
Fat (total)	6.92 g
Saturated fat	0.92 g
Cholesterol	23.76 mg
Sodium	148.63 mg

Sam's Mulled Christmas Cider

1 gallon apple juice (the "not from concentrate" is good, and real apple cider is best!)
4 whole cloves
4 whole allspice
Half of a crushed or chopped nutmeg
2 cinnamon sticks
Put all in a pan and heat on medium until almost to a boil.
Reduce to low heat for 2–3 hours.
Serve hot in mugs.
Optional: This can be made into an alcoholic beverage by adding dry red wine.

Servings: 6 (6 ounces each)
What's in one serving?

Calories	90.87
Protein	0.4 g
Carbohydrates	22.67 g
Dietary fiber	0.04 g
Fat (total)	0.02 g
Saturated fat	0.01 g
Cholesterol	0 mg
Sodium	18.80 mg

POTLUCKS AND PICNICS

Mustard Slaw* (see pages 244–245)

Servings: 20

What's in one serving?

Calories	127.49
Protein	3.53 g
Carbohydrates	27.05 g
Dietary fiber	5.05 g
Fat (total)	2.04 g
Saturated fat	0.83 g
Cholesterol	2.53 mg
Sodium	5.22 mg

Lalita's Friendship Brownies

This is a fun recipe to take along as a housewarming, thank-you, or any kind of gift. These brownies can be made right away or the dry ingredients saved for another time.

You need a 1-quart glass container with a tight-fitting lid. Into this container, you carefully add layers of

1 cup plus 2 T all-purpose flour

⅔ cup packed brown sugar

¾ tsp salt

⅔ cup sugar

1 tsp baking powder

⅓ cup baking cocoa

½ cup semisweet chocolate chips

½ cup chopped walnuts

Do not mix! Give this gift to a friend or neighbor with this recipe. When covered tightly and stored in cool dry place, this is good for up to 6 months.

When it's time to prepare the brownies, you'll need

3 eggs

⅔ cup vegetable oil

1 tsp vanilla

In a bowl, beat the eggs, oil, and vanilla. Slowly add the brownie mix from the glass container. Stir well. Spread into a greased 9-inch square baking pan. Bake at 350° for about 35 minutes or until a toothpick stuck in the center comes out clean.

Cool on a wire rack.

Servings: 16 brownies
What's in one serving (1 brownie)?

Calories	212.83
Protein	3.42 g
Carbohydrates	20.48 g
Dietary fiber	1.07 g
Fat (total)	14.20 g
Saturated fat	2.34 g
Cholesterol	35.06 mg
Sodium	154.26 mg

Mustard Slaw

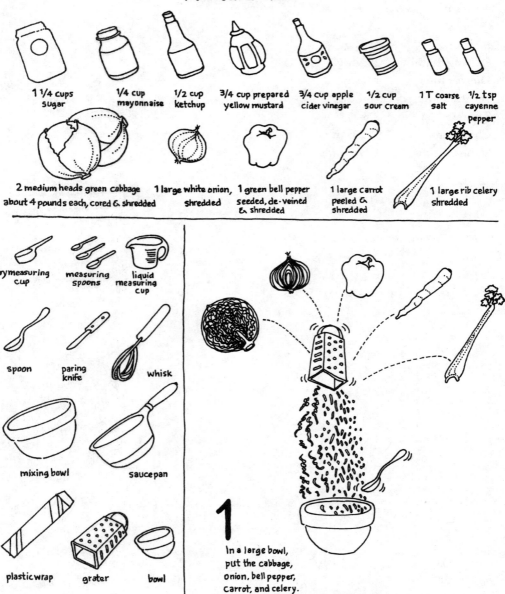

1 1/4 cups sugar

1/4 cup mayonnaise

1/2 cup ketchup

3/4 cup prepared yellow mustard

3/4 cup apple cider vinegar

1/2 cup sour cream

1 T coarse salt

1/2 tsp cayenne pepper

2 medium heads green cabbage about 4 pounds each, cored & shredded

1 large white onion, shredded

1 green bell pepper seeded, de-veined & shredded

1 large carrot peeled & shredded

1 large rib celery shredded

dry measuring cup

measuring spoons

liquid measuring cup

spoon

paring knife

whisk

mixing bowl

sauce pan

plastic wrap

grater

bowl

1

In a large bowl, put the cabbage, onion, bell pepper, carrot, and celery. Mix everything together.

2

In a small saucepan add the vinegar,
mustard, ketchup, sour cream, mayo,
salt, and cayenne.

3

Bring this mixture to a boil
and whisk frequently.

4

Pour it over the cabbage mixture.
Add the sugar and stir more
to mix it up well.

5

Cover the bowl with plastic wrap
(or a "hotel hat" – a new shower cap
works great!) and put it in the
refrigerator.

6

When you serve it, have a bowl
of roughly chopped dry roasted
peanuts to sprinkle on the top.

Servings: 20

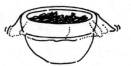
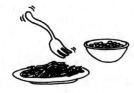

FREEZER BEES/HARVEST PUT-UPS

Vegetable or Chicken Pot Pies

You can host a Pot Pie Party! Have some people assemble the filling and others prepare the dough and line either large or individual foil dishes. See Jim's Apple Pie on page 236 for an easy pie dough recipe. The pie dough can line the entire pan plus the top or just the top.

Filling:
1 cup chopped onions
1 cup chopped red bell pepper
2 cloves garlic, minced
2½ cups vegetable broth (or chicken stock if you're doing a chicken version)
2 T olive oil
2 cups peeled, small cubed potatoes
1 cup sliced carrots
(2 cups cooked cubed skinless chicken for chicken version)
1½ tsp dried rosemary
½ tsp dried thyme
1 tsp dried tarragon
¼ tsp salt
¼ tsp pepper
1 cup frozen green peas, thawed
3 tablespoons flour
¼ cup chopped fresh parsley

Heat 2 tablespoons olive oil and sauté onions, red pepper, and garlic. Sauté until softened, about 4 minutes.

Add 2 cups broth (or chicken stock), potatoes, carrots, rosemary, thyme, salt, and pepper. (Add 2 cups chicken for chicken version.)

Bring to a boil. Turn to low, cover, and simmer about 10–12 minutes.

In a separate bowl, mix 3 T flour with ½ cup broth, add tarragon, mix until smooth. Add to vegetable mixture, cook until thickened. Add parsley. Option: Sauté mushrooms, onions, and garlic in butter and olive oil, sprinkle it all with flour, then add the liquid.

Stir in peas, cook 3 more minutes.

Scoop mixture into foil baking dishes (individual ones are good, also medium sized for 2–4 servings). Insert each pie when complete into a zip-lock freezer bag or secure the bag tightly and freeze on level surface in the freezer. Once frozen, you can stack them. In the meantime, don't forget to bake one to reward everyone for the hard work!

When ready to bake, pull out the number you need and bake at 350° for approximately 45 minutes. Insert a fork to test for heat in the center.

Servings: Makes several (depending on what size pies are made)
What's in one serving? (filling)

Calories	341.10
Protein	20.27 g
Carbohydrates	30.04 g
Dietary fiber	2.91 g
Fat (total)	15.25 g
Saturated fat	4.80 g
Cholesterol	47.53 mg
Sodium	383.80 mg

Freezer Stock-up Soup

This is good to make in a big batch, then freeze in smaller or individual serving containers. Try out other soup recipes and freeze for reheating later.

1 cup cheese spread (e.g., Cheez Whiz)
1 can (10 fl. oz./284 ml) chicken broth (or mix from soup base powder)
1 tsp Italian seasoning
1 lb boneless chicken pieces, bite-sized
1 cup small, bite-sized pasta such as penne
4 chopped carrots (½ inch chunks)
1 cup sliced celery
1 chopped onion
2 cups water

In a pot, add 1 T olive oil at medium high. Add 1 lb boneless chicken pieces, bite-sized. Stir until chicken is cooked through. Drain.
Add vegetables and stir; cook 3–5 minutes.
Add second can of chicken broth, 2 cups water, and Italian seasonings.
Bring to a boil.
Add pasta and simmer 10–12 mins. Pasta should be tender.
Stir in cheese spread until well blended.
Cool soup thoroughly before ladling into small, freezer-proof containers with tight lids. Label containers with soup name and date.
Thaw in refrigerator as needed. Reheat on high in microwave or in a pan on the stovetop.
Note: You can omit the chicken if desired, or add other vegetables such as chopped red pepper, zucchini. Experiment!

Servings: 8 (1 cup each)
What's in one serving?
Calories   202.79
Protein   10.76 g
Carbohydrates   16.95 g
Dietary fiber   1.96 g
Fat (total)   10.34 g
Saturated fat   5.88 g
Cholesterol   36.27 mg
Sodium   852.56 mg

Easy Rhubarb Jelly Jam

6 cups rhubarb, remove strings and leaves, chop into small cubes
5 cups sugar
1 tin crushed pineapple
Cook 20 minutes. Take off heat. Add 2 boxes of strawberry Jell-O. Stir well.
Pack while hot in sterilized jars and seal.
Yield: approximately 10 8-oz jars

What's in one serving (1 T)?
Calories   31.85
Protein   0.15 g
Carbohydrates   8.10 g
Dietary fiber   0.10 g
Fat (total)   0.01g
Saturated fat   0.00 g
Cholesterol   0 mg
Sodium   2.81 mg

Faith's Easy Pickles

9 cups sliced unpeeled cucumbers (can also use English cucumbers)
1 cup sliced onions
Mix together: 1 cup white vinegar, 2 cups white sugar, 2 T pickling salt, 1tsp celery
    seed. Pour mixture over cucumber/onions.
Store in glass or Tupperware dish (not aluminum); cover and keep in the refrigerator.
Let stand at least overnight and use as needed.
Keeps up to one week.
Optional: Can also add sliced slightly blanched carrots, cauliflower pieces, or asparagus
    pieces. Could also add cloves of raw peeled garlic, ¼ cup diced red pepper, and fresh
    or dried dill, 1 tsp red pepper flakes for heat.

Servings: 20
What's in one serving?

Calories   90.46
Protein   1.23 g
Carbohydrates   22.03 g
Dietary fiber   0.61 g
Fat (total)   0.18 g
Saturated fat   0.03 g
Cholesterol   0 mg
Sodium   710.91 mg

My Recipe for _____

Ingredients

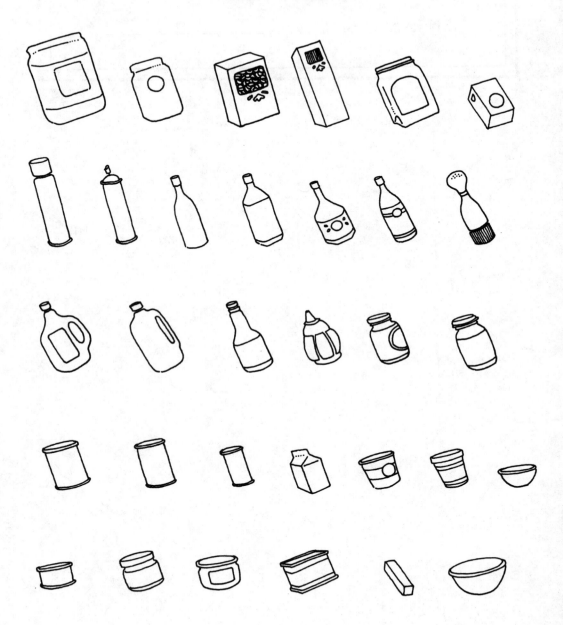

Ingredients

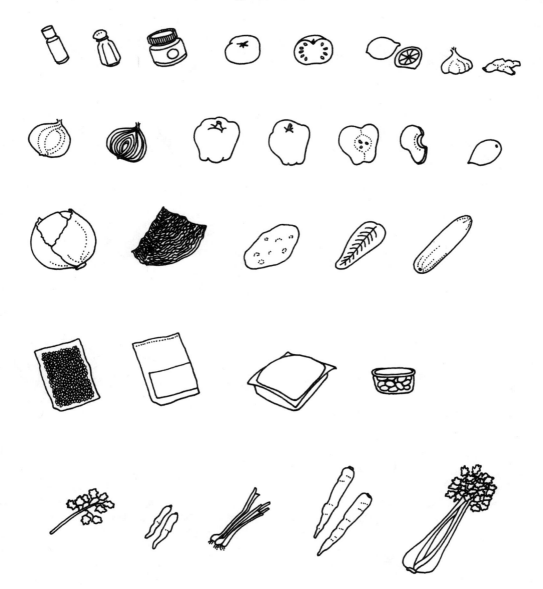

Dishes and Utensils

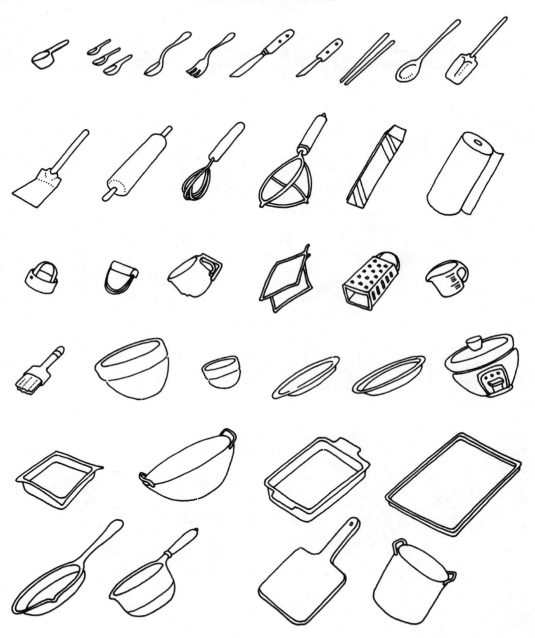

Tidbits by Category

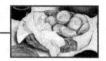

Throughout this book, tidbits on several aspects of dining have been given in most chapters. Here, these tidbits are organized by category and chapter for ease of reading or if you are particularly interested in one type. Note that not every chapter has tidbits or the same number of tidbits in each category.

SAFETY AND HEALTH

Chapter 2

If people aren't hungry, they shouldn't be forced to eat. People shouldn't feel forced to clean their plates. Offer the possibility of putting food away to warm up later.

Allergies and asthma can produce a variety of unpleasant sensations. Coughing, sneezing, and gasping can cause serious problems such as aspiration (inhaling small amounts of food and liquid into the lungs) at mealtime. Be aware of how to minimize these difficulties; talk to the person, her family, and her caregivers to learn strategies that work.

Chapter 4

Hot dogs, candy, nuts, and grapes account for almost half of all choking deaths in young children (Harris, Baker, Smith, & Harris, 1984). Soft, loosely textured foods (such as bread) that become compressed upon swallowing are responsible for approximately 15% of such deaths (Dailey, 1983); this probably occurs more commonly in older children and adults with multiple disabilities. Danger foods can be ground and mixed with a little gravy. Without gravy or other moisture, ground food can often be sucked into the windpipe when breathing in. Grapes should be cut in half. There are companies that make puréed spread; you just add water and mix. Peanut butter, too, can be made edible by mixing in jelly or even soft tofu. Soft spreads such as peanut butter without jelly and marshmallow cream should be avoided (Sobsey & Thuppal, 1996).

Always wash your hands carefully with soap and water before doing any care of someone's tube.

Chapter 9

If you decide to light a candle for more atmosphere at the dining table, remember that candles with strong odors may not only interfere with the taste pleasures but also may cause respiratory problems, so get nonscented candles.

If you find out that an individual has swallowing difficulties, a powder additive, available for purchase in some grocery stores and pharmacies, can be added by spoonfuls to liquid to make it easier to swallow. It can be used with any liquid and can be taken anywhere. If you are at a restaurant and don't want to draw undue attention to the can, take a small bit in a discreet plastic bag. Add it to anything and tell anyone who asks that it is protein powder or a strength supplement!

Chapter 14

If you are planning to dine with a person who has food texture restrictions, such as the need for a puréed-only diet or the need to have all liquids thickened because of difficulty swallowing, perhaps this is a perfect chance for you both to try those health food shakes and smoothies at juice stores.

Appendix A

Make sure people know how to use oven mitts. And what do you do if the smoke detector goes off? It can be quite startling and scary for someone who doesn't know what it means!

Wash your hands often when handling and preparing food, and before eating.

Make sure to keep raw poultry such as chicken separate from other foods. Wash cutting boards, utensils, and hands after handling raw chicken and before using those utensils again.

Remember, any time you're preparing food, you must wash your hands before you start. Use soap and warm water. Turn away from food, utensils, and work areas if you have to sneeze or cough, then wash your hands again. Remember to use a potholder or oven mitt to take hot pans out of the oven.

 GOOD IDEA

Chapter 2

Have a manageable number of food items during a meal. Some people can be overwhelmed with too many choices and decisions.

Not all people with disabilities will need physical assistance with eating.

Pay attention to the table setting. For some people who have perception and visual difficulties, a white plate, a clear glass, silver cutlery, and a white napkin on a white tablecloth may "disappear." Try arranging light-colored foods such as potatoes and pasta on a dark-colored plate, for example, so there is a contrast.

Chapter 4

If the person has significant disabilities, help her relax before mealtime begins. Talk about what you're doing, what you'll be eating, and when. Imagine what it might feel like to come to the table with tense muscles and no knowledge of what you'll be expected to eat.

Chapter 6

Everyone likes to go places where people know their name. Get to know local shopkeepers. Model friendly and courteous behavior. Always involve the person with the disability in the exchange, whether it's a chat in the aisle or making the purchases at the till.

Investigate neighborhood teas and potlucks. They're a great opportunity for getting to know the neighbors and an excuse to get cooking.

Here is a great tip for people who use Velcro symbols. Try a wall-mounted communication board made up of a 2-foot by 2-foot carpet runner. You can get one at Home Depot for about $4. It's glued to the wall with contact cement and various symbols, like which restaurant sounds good for supper, and can be backed with Velcro and peeled off the board when it's time to make a choice.

Some microwaves come with pre-programmed buttons with pictures of the food along with the name to ensure appropriate cooking time. Stick the bag of popcorn in, close the door and hit the popcorn button.

Outside picnics are great if spilling is a concern. The birds and squirrels will thank you for it. Indoor "carpet picnics" are also great if sitting in a chair is challenging. Do it just for fun, and no need to worry about ants.

Asking for help in the corner market or grocery store is a good way to involve people in their local community. Remember to include everyone in the conversation so everyone interacts in whatever way they can.

Always be respectful of personal space.

Chapter 9

The Golden Rule of "Do unto others as you would have them do unto you" applies to your dining experiences.

Try playing some nice music while you're cooking and eating.

If you are looking for an accessible restaurant in your area, try a web search. Type in "accessible dining" and the name of your city. It will pull up a varied list of places and their accessibility features reviewed by people with disabilities.

Turn off the cell phone and television for mealtimes.

Chapter 10

In western countries, there are interfaith, ecumenical, and specific faith networks that connect people who are committed to inclusion of people with disabilities and their families. Those include the Religion and Spirituality Division of the AAMR, the Christian Council for Persons with Disabilities, the National Apostolate for Inclusion Ministries, the National Catholic Partnership with People with Disabilities, and the Religion and Disability Program of the National Organization on Disability.

Chapter 11

Are people welcome in the kitchen? One residential director we know makes it a practice to invite people into the kitchen to help with muffins and cookies. If they don't feel like helping, they might enjoy a cup of tea or coffee, and it's visiting time while the kitchen is warm and wonderful with baking.

When making food with large groups, split the tasks. If making an entire pie or four dozen cookies is too much for one session, try mixing the ingredients on one occasion. Pop the dough in the freezer. Thaw the dough in preparation for the next time you get together.

Pre-prepare and package meals in separate containers; store in the refrigerator or freezer and with reheating instructions. This can make for easy and more independent cooking.

For people whose physical disabilities keep them from being neat eaters, how about hosting a toga party? Nobody worries about spills and messes if everybody's wearing a sheet!

Talk with someone who has a disability in the same tone of voice as you would with anyone else. Avoid the temptation to singsong or end all of your sentences in an upswing as if they are questions.

When planning a shopping trip to find the ingredients for a meal to prepare together, give someone who has little or no language skills a chance to help prepare the list. Spread a sale flier out and suggest he circle some of the items you need. Take the flier along to the store and hunt down the circled items together. If a grocery shopping experience is a bit overwhelming, try a small convenience store. Or go with a list so you can contain the experience but still get out and about.

Pre-cut and washed vegetables and salad fixings are available in the produce section, or you can make your own ahead of time and store in an airtight bag. For beginning cooks, or people who want to get to the finish line more quickly, the end result is more apparent sooner. Adding extra tomatoes, zucchini, green peppers, and radishes to a bowl of ready-made salad still creates a sense of achievement quickly!

Ready to pull apart/cut-and-bake cookies, bread, pizza crust, dinner rolls, and biscuits are available in most dairy or bakery sections of the grocery store. These can offer a sense of immediate accomplishment. Cookie dough from scratch can be made ahead and frozen in portions, ready to pull out for an afternoon of baking.

Chapter 12

Make a visual shopping list. Clip pictures of items for purchase from grocery fliers or magazines. Save the labels from the food containers to use on the next shopping trip. This can also be helpful for someone with limited language or speech skills.

Chapter 14

Too much parsley in the container garden? Cut it back low on the stalk and tie up the excess bunches for drying. It's a great project to do at the kitchen table. Hang bunches in a warm, dry place. Wait about a week for them to dry completely or you can leave them hanging about the kitchen! You can do this with thyme, tarragon, sage, basil, and bay leaves, too.

If you are going out to eat, try to pick up a menu a few days before you go. You can discuss the menu items and make food choices beforehand without the distractions of the busy restaurant environment. This may eliminate some stress, if this is an issue. This also gives you and your dining partner an opportunity to discuss some of the situations that you may have to negotiate at the restaurant, and you can practice before you go.

 FOOD FOR THOUGHT

Chapter 2

Many people find the question of bib use to be a quandary. On the one hand, some people who have difficulty managing food and eating have found bibs helpful in protecting their clothing. On the other hand, the worry is that bibs detract from someone's dignity. Clothing protectors or aprons look less infantile. For anyone who's not an infant, avoid cartoon characters and juvenile designs. When helping someone eat, don't use the bib to wipe the person's mouth. That's what a napkin is for. And never leave a soiled bib, clothing protector, or apron on someone after a meal.

In our society, it's acceptable to cut food at the table for small children. But if you or your meal partner still requires the food to be cut up but would be embarrassed by this assistance, why not do the cutting in the kitchen before presenting it at the table? If you're dining out, make the request of the server when you order. An adult with dignity intact can manage a sliced chicken breast or a de-boned and sliced pork chop.

Chapter 4

Have you ever been seated in a restaurant only to have the server ignore you? When he or she finally does arrive, water glasses are slammed down and specials mumbled in a way you don't understand. Did you get the feeling the server would rather you just got up and left and quit bothering him? Contrast that with your best dining experience. Mealtimes can feel like a frantic assembly line for people with disabilities. Remember to make the experience a memorable one.

Never talk past the person you are sharing mealtime with. Talk to that person. If you are talking with other people, too, make sure no one is left out. Explain what you're talking about, what the other person is saying, and involve them, even though the topic of conversation may not be fully understood by all.

Think of the person with a disability in terms of his or her chronological age as much as possible. Because helping someone eat is generally what we do with babies and young children, there is a danger of treating a person with a disability as an infant, stripping away self-esteem and falling prey to the old myth of the eternal child. Be sensitive.

Think about what the home smells like. Are there institutional cleaners and odors, or are you welcomed with the aromas of baking, homemade dinner, and dessert in the oven?

The Dining with Dignity program at Holy Name Hospital, Teaneck, New Jersey, was established by the Dysphagia Interdisciplinary Committee with the Food and Nutrition Services Department. There's a mouthful. With great success, they began serving puréed food that is reshaped to look like the real thing. Gelled cookies and carrot "coins" offer visual stimulation and texture to make eating more pleasurable.

Children with disabilities need support to go through the messy developmental stage of exploring taste, texture, early grasp, and control of their environment. Sometimes older people with disabilities have missed this opportunity for discovery. We say, better late than never! Put down a sheet for a picnic. Let everyone get messy. Encourage an older person with a disability to explore what food feels like, tastes like, how funny it can be when you throw it. No one should go through life without at least one food fight.

If someone uses a tube at mealtime, the need for the mealtime experience still exists. Some people enjoy the sensory element of taste and enjoy something in their mouth. Some people are able to taste and spit; you can help this to happen discreetly.

To share mealtimes with someone who makes use of a tube for food intake, learn a bit about him or her. There are nasogastric tubes (NG-tubes) that are inserted into one nostril, down the throat, and into the stomach. The stomach end has a rounded piece that allows liquid nourishment to flow into the stomach. Gastrostomy tubes (G-tubes) require surgical placement and deliver nourishment directly to the stomach. Remember that enjoyment of the mealtime experience is a lot more than just the insertion of nutrients!

Consider what you have in common with the person you are dining with in addition to the food you are eating. This can make for better mealtime conversation. Are you both Trekkies? Maybe you've been to the same places.

For some people, mealtime may be the best chance during the day to spend time with someone who will focus on them completely.

Chapter 6

Remember that someone may have had a "bad food experience" in the past. Perhaps they were forced to eat something they didn't like. Don't force people to eat something.

Is the food being served to someone with a disability something you would enjoy or would just tolerate?

Add color to meals. Cauliflower, mashed potatoes, and steamed whitefish might be nutritious, but how blah it looks! Color stimulates interest and visual enjoyment of foods.

Offer choices about when to eat, how the table might be decorated, and if the meal should be served up at the stove or family-style at the table.

Never use food as a reward. That doesn't mean one should never mark a special occasion with a celebration dinner or a chocolate shake. But to use food as a motivational tool to entice someone to do chores or behave in certain ways isn't a great idea. People are not pets. Similarly, denying food puts mealtime in the awkward position of punishment rather than enjoyable activity.

Do you have snacks available in the cupboard or fridge that people can help themselves to if they feel the munchies coming on? This is an adult privilege most of us take for granted, but something that may be denied to an adult with a disability.

Make a conscious effort to leave your "teacher" self behind from time to time. Let things go. Let there be times when you just enjoy each other. We call them "No Nag Days."

Chapter 9

Learn what kinds of foods make people happy. Is there a special birthday cake that brings back wonderful childhood memories?

Come to the kitchen or the table ready to be emotionally devoted to being with that person for this time. Your mealtime companion deserves your total attention.

The grocery store, farmer's market, and flower shop are all treasure troves of sensory experiences. Take time to savor the sights, sounds, smells and textures. Make it a hands-on experience.

Chapter 10

Wondering about mealtimes in different religions and faiths? Visit http://www.familyvillage.wisc.edu/, and click on House of Worship, which has related resources, materials, and organizations. Also try http://www.qualitymall.org and the Religion and Spirituality Division, AAMR at: http://www.aamrreligion.org.

Chapter 11

Remember what you enjoy at mealtime: easy conversation, good humor, nice music, a calm atmosphere, and tasty food. Some people with disabilities may take some time to see this as a pleasant alternative to the rushed, noisy, overstimulated, staff-driven experience they may be used to having.

Are people living in the home encouraged to clear after a meal? Many people feel proud to help tidy up. Always be ready with compliments and thanks for the help. Everyone needs to feel like they are doing for themselves.

Do people know how to use the microwave? A simple chart with a food item and the time for cooking or warming up can be an easy guide to kitchen independence.

Anticipation is more than half the fun of a meal. Do you plan for Thanksgiving feast the day before? Chances are, you're thinking about it for at least weeks ahead of time. Help someone with a disability enjoy the flood of feelings and sensations that lead up to your time together.

Do you remember how undignified you felt when your mom would pull an old tissue out of her purse and wipe your face in public? Or worse, when she would lick her thumb and try to scrub something off of your face? Please don't do that to anyone!

Chapter 12

Arrange for people living in your residential agency to invite family and friends for dinner now and then. Make sure people can show off their skills and talents in the kitchen.

Chapter 14

Tomatoes and herbs are easy to grow in a small container garden. Build the garden to meet the person's needs. Does she use a wheelchair, or would bending over to care for the plant be difficult? Maybe a raised container would allow better access.

If a person is resistant to eating, stop chasing the person's mouth with a spoon or pestering them with a breadstick. Give the person some space.

Consider the person's ability or inability to switch gears if the meal consists of an item that can be eaten with the hands, such as a sandwich, and another that requires a fork, such as a side of potato salad. Serving items separately might be easier.

If someone is distressed at mealtime, survey the environment. Are too many choices being offered? Are the colors disturbing? Is there an issue with the people close by? Is the food not to their liking? Is someone staring? Is there a table leg in the way? Are you asking the person to sit in someone else's chair? Are you truly "with" the person, or distracted by something?

People with disabilities, especially intellectual disabilities, are plagued by the myth of the eternal child. Ask adults what they like to be called; don't assume childish versions are the preference just because other people use them. Bob shouldn't become "Bobby," Jim isn't "Jimmy," Kimberley isn't "Kimmy." And think about what to say if others insist on calling someone with a disability "honey," "sweetheart," or "sweetie." Often, strangers will do this in an effort to be friendly, but it crosses the line of intimacy.

Mealtime can be a great social equalizer. If someone with a disability requires medications at mealtime, be sensitive and discreet. If dining in public or even at home, for that matter, use an attractive pillbox that could pass as a compact or glasses case. You are both diners having a nice meal, not nurse and patient.

 POSITIONING

Chapter 2

Some people with cerebral palsy who have more muscle involvement can expend a lot of energy in the daily struggle to control muscle coordination. Learn the person's preferences as to how much support to receive. Something you think is an important task, like eating unassisted, may be too exhausting for the person to manage for a whole meal.

If you are helping someone to eat, pay close attention to the person's breathing patterns. A forkful of food shouldn't be presented during an inhale or exhale, but rather, just before either.

Make sure you are at the same level as the person or slightly lower when helping him eat so he isn't looking upward and hyper-extending his neck.

If someone cannot physically manage to wipe his or her own mouth during the meal, ask if you can assist. Don't swoop in, push the person's head back, and wipe. Without fuss and with dignity, ask if you may help, and then say what you're going to do. Then wipe with a napkin—firmly but gently—and start at the side of the person's mouth.

When you are assisting someone who requires a lot of support to eat his or meal, you are, in essence, replacing the person's hand to eat (Zgola, personal communication, 2003). Sitting kitty-corner is useful for comfortable contact and hand movement.

One's mouth and hands work better when one's trunk and shoulders have a firm base of support. A footrest helps. So does a lap tray or a table; it's not just a place to put the plate but a helpful foundation for elbows to stabilize the neck and head.

Use your own body to give support to someone if needed to help the person get into a comfortable position for eating. Each person is unique, so a pillow or wedge that works well for one person may not work for someone else.

Pay attention to how a person is sitting for a meal. Sitting straight and comfortably with feet on the floor makes it easier for someone to use his or her arms and to swallow properly.

Chapter 14

Change positions during a task such as peeling potatoes, making salad, or even eating. For someone with limited mobility who may need support to shift positions, awareness and assistance from the person they're with is appreciated. Having pins and needles in the arms and legs isn't a fun way to finish off a meal!

If you are taking a person with a significant disability out to eat and you don't know him well, take along a snapshot of the person in his preferred position for eating. Maybe you can jot some reminder tips on the back of the photograph that will help make the experience safe and comfortable for everyone.

 ## GADGETS

Chapter 2

If adapted utensils are needed, respect the person's age and dignity. Look for the most age-appropriate options. A Winnie-the-Pooh tippy cup is fine for a 3-year-old, but what does it say about a 30-year-old?

Use clear or translucent cups with a person who needs assistance to drink so you can see when the fluid reaches his mouth. Iced tea up the nose isn't pleasant.

What can you do if you're cooking, baking, or eating a meal and the bowl or dish won't stay still? Cut out a piece of Dycem, a nonsticky sheeting that grips on both sides. Dycem comes in small pieces, as place mats, or in rolls so you can cut to the desired length and shape. You can try plastic cupboard lining, too; it's in the kitchen supply aisle of the supermarket. Put it underneath while you're stirring or eating to keep the bowl or plate from sliding away. A word of caution: Dycem and other nonskid materials can be made of latex, and some people have an allergy to this. Plastic liners are a good way to avoid reactions, but in general, do pay attention to skin allergies as well as to food allergies.

Chapter 4

Do you know someone who has trouble reaching and grabbing? Reachers with grasping ends operated by a simple trigger mechanism help people reach for things on the ground and on lower shelves. Emphasize to someone with a disability that, when shopping, it is still important to ask store employees, family members, and friends for help in reaching heavier items up high.

Do you know someone who likes to bake? If you find those crank sifters too hard to manage, battery-operated flour sifters eliminate the need to turn the crank.

Try using electric can openers that sit on the counter. If cans are hard to open, all this requires is that you hold the can up to the magnet and push a button.

Have trouble holding onto utensils? Velcro bands with a pocket at the palm of the hand (sometimes called a "universal cuff") can be used to insert a spoon or a fork and can be wrapped around a hand.

Bendable utensils and jar and bottle openers make handling objects easier.

Some spoons have sharp edges. One of the best spoons for some people with disabilities is the type with a vinyl covering to avoid injury. White is the most common but tends to stain from tomato and curry sauces. Red is a little startling. Try navy blue. Avoid baby utensils; ask at a kitchen supply store if less juvenile looking ones can be ordered.

Chapter 6

Many kitchen appliances now come with independence-giving safety features, such as automatic shut-off kettles and coffee makers, cool-touch toasters, and bladeless electric can openers.

For someone who has difficulty scooping, try a swivel spoon. These spoons have a swivel mechanism that helps individuals without much control in their wrists to eat their own meals without dumping food.

Chapter 9

Does someone not have the hand strength or grasp to manage slicing cheese? Some cutting boards come with spikes to stabilize food while cutting without the need to use both hands.

Having trouble making bread "stay still" while you're making sandwiches or dressing up toast in the morning? Breadboards come with corner guards so the bread can be secured in the corner and it won't slide around.

A one-handed rocker knife or ulu makes for easier cutting. No need to saw.

Weighted utensils and cutlery make it easier for someone with limited hand control or tremors.

Chapter 11

For someone who can scoop but can't quite turn the utensil into the mouth, there are spoons available that are angled to the right or left of the stem to point directly at the mouth. These are also easily made by picking up some lightweight utensils at your local thrift or consignment store and bending them to fit your needs.

Cut-away cups allow the cup to be tipped up high enough without the person tipping their head back. Cut-away cups can be made from dishwasher-safe plastic. Make your own by cutting and sanding out a piece, or order from catalogues.

Chapter 14

Commercial plate guards that help keep food from being pushed off can be orthopedic-looking. Consider finding dishes that have narrow rims along the inside. The design serves the same purpose without drawing attention.

Special scrubbers with handles are available that can make it easier for someone with little hand control to wash dishes.

Appendix A

Cookbooks can be awkward to handle. Buy a plate stand or book display rack at a kitchen supply store. They're cheap and you can prop open the book (including this one!) to the pages you want, for hands-free reference.

MISCELLANEOUS

The following Tidbits were not listed in any chapter but are still helpful ideas related to nourishing connections with people with and without disabilities at mealtime.

 GOOD IDEA

If going to the grocery store is just too much stimulation, most large chain grocery stores have an option to order your groceries online and have them sent. You can shop by the pictures on the computer screen and have them delivered.

Standing for long periods in the kitchen can be tiring and stressful. Think of ways tasks such as chopping vegetables, mixing ingredients, throwing a salad together, and washing dishes can be done while sitting rather than standing.

Some grocery stores also have pick-up and drop-off service available upon request. They will pick you up at your house or apartment and take you to the market, then take you home when you are done. Some supermarkets have delivery available even if you don't order the groceries on line. Just ask the customer service person about the services available.

A miracle invention: ready-to-bake lasagna noodles!

Start a cookie exchange. Each person bakes a dozen or so of his favorite kind, then brings them and copies of the recipe to a get-together. Everyone gets to take home an assortment and new recipes to try.

Have a harvest bee in the fall. There are simple jam recipes that make for a fun afternoon in the kitchen. Decorated jars of colorful preserves make great gifts that fill the giver with pride.

FOOD FOR THOUGHT

Why not try having breakfast in bed one morning?

Organize an ethnic potluck.

Invite a gathering of friends and ask each to bring along enough copies of a favorite recipe for everyone. This could be the beginning of a great Potluck Club.

Human beings like results. We want feedback. Sometimes a person with a disability responds in a way we're not used to or don't expect. We may make assumptions about that which lead us to behave in ways that discourage communication. Think of your own tone of voice, facial expression, and body language. What messages are you giving?

Transitions from one activity to another can be stressful for some people. An abrupt, unannounced change can leave a person disoriented and confused. Try to help someone prepare and get used to the idea of leaving one activity to start another. Give the person information of what, when, and where. A visual cue, such as a picture, may help. We all look forward to something we like to do.

All people have some aversions to certain food textures. Some people don't like tomatoes, mushrooms, creamed corn, or couscous. Be aware of your own preferences so that it's not strange for you to hear what foods other people cannot handle. And be sure to always ask people about their likes and dislikes. That way you can find similarities and make a pact with a friend early on to never serve cow tongue!

We know of a retired director of nursing who became a group home manager in a small town. She took great pride in wearing her nurse's uniform in the home and whenever she accompanied the women out for grocery shopping or even a meal downtown.

Unfortunately, she merely added to the medical model myth that people with disabilities are sick.

A life-long quandary for people with disabilities is a need for support and assistance, but also the need to be seen as growing, learning human beings. By all means have fun together. Laugh. Joke around. But don't belittle the attempts made by someone who is learning. Pointing out mistakes, especially putting them on display for others, can be painful. To be called "cute" and "funny" when you're trying hard to be seen and respected as an adult isn't that amusing if it becomes a habit.